Lectures on Localization in Diseases of the
Brain
Delivered At The Faculte De Medecine, Paris,
1875
©1878
By
J.M. Charcot

AUTHOR'S PREFACE.

THE exposition of the principles underlying the doctrine of cerebral localization seems to have now become a necessary chapter of introduction to the practical study of diseases of the brain.

In the Lectures which Dr. Fowler has kindly taken the pains to submit to the appreciation of our American *confrères*, I have selected, as occasion required, information furnished by normal anatomy, experimental physiology, and clinical observation, illustrated by minute and methodical examination of organic lesions.

I have always given precedence, however, to the last-mentioned order of testimony, convinced that, although normal anatomy and experimental physiology may serve to indicate the true direction; still, clinical and pathological research is necessary (in case of the human subject) to a final judgment and to the *furnishing of proof.*

I shall consider it as a great honor if my book should be favorably received in a country where instructors in neural pathology are represented by scientists such as my friend W. Mitchell, and various others whom I might enumerate.

In any event, I cannot sufficiently thank Dr. Fowler for the care which he has bestowed upon the translation, and I unhesitatingly say that it appears to me a model, both of scrupulous exactitude in rendition of the original meaning, and as a clear and unexceptionable style of English.

J. M. CHARCOT.

PARIS, Oct. 26, 1878.

TRANSLATOR'S PREFACE.

No excuse is required for contributions to medical literature which are calculated to increase exactitude of expression, ideas, and knowledge, thereby assisting to elevate medical Art to the higher plane of Science.

These lectures are a bold example of that cast, as indeed are all of Charcot's teachings and writings.

It is too late to introduce our distinguished author to the medical profession, for wherever medicine is taught as a science his works are already known and prized, and have been translated into nearly every modern language. This, however, is the first volume which has been published in this country.

Charcot's superstructures are always built with great care and reserve upon the secure basis of induction, though he is none the less resplendent in the rich harvest of deduction which naturally follows.

The translator cannot refrain from expressing his conviction that the perfecting of medical knowledge depends mainly upon those investigators of which Charcot is so brilliant and so sound a representative.

New York, July, 1878.

CONTENTS.

TENTH LECTURE.

ELEVENTH LECTURE.

TWELFTH LECTURE.

LECTURES UPON LOCALIZATION

IN

DISEASES OF THE BRAIN.

FIRST LECTURE.

LOCALIZATION IN CEREBRAL DISEASES.

Summary :—Preamble.—Apparent Aridity of the Study of Cerebral Localization.—Principles of Localization.—The Encephalon in a Morphological Point of View.—Necessity of an Exact Nomenclature. —Topography of the Convolutions. — Importance of Comparative Anatomy.—Convolutions of the Brain of the Monkey; Frontal, Parietal, and Sphenoidal Lobes.—Psycho-motor Centres.—Differences in the Composition of the Gray Substance in the Various Regions of the Brain.

GENTLEMEN :

I. We will devote the first part of this year's course to the *anatomico-pathological study* of the encephalon. Every one in an audience of medical practitioners will recognize the importance of this subject. But, with some, the lack of an attractive exterior has given it an unfortunate reputation ; in this particular I hope to inspire you with a different sentiment. Through a method already often employed, aided also by a certain amount of patience and perseverance—and that will not be lacking on my part, I assure you—I think we shall accomplish this task without undue fatigue or difficulty.

To avoid leading you unprepared into the domain where

we shall journey together, I will make, by way of an introduction, some observations concerning general facts, the application of which facts will be obvious at each subsequent
step.

I have little faith in the value of generalities when unaccompanied by their material substructure, and especially as
concerns pathological anatomy. I will therefore supply such
groundwork by furnishing a certain number of actual illustra-
tions. These examples will be taken from the most important chapter in encephalic pathology, that treating of *localization in cerebral diseases*.

Various reasons have decided my choice of subject. In
the first place, it is one of those fields of inquiry where the
advantage of associating clinical with anatomico-pathological
studies is most conspicuously evident; upon the principles of
cerebral localization is founded that which may be called
regional diagnosis of encephalic diseases, that ideal toward
the realization of which, in this special section of pathology,
should be directed all the efforts of clinical teaching.

Then, again, the question of cerebral localization has entered a new phase, and is now enlisting world-wide attention.

We should not make undue sacrifices to fashion, but on
the other hand we must not undervalue the attractions and
the new facts presented by recent investigations.

In a thesis offered at the last *concours d'aggrégation de
médecine*, this interesting chapter has been handled with
great ability by my friend and old pupil, Dr. Lépine, *agrégé*
of that faculty. I shall be happy to utilize the delicately dis-
criminated observations which abound in that work, and to
turn to profit the wealth of erudition which the author has
there accumulated.

It is understood, of course, that in these preliminary lectures
we can give only a free outline. The subjects which I shall
introduce should be resumed later, submitted to a more profound study, and examined in their most minute details.

II.—Long explanations are unnecessary to convey what is
meant by *localization* in cerebral physiology and pathology.

The term has long since become a common one, and its meaning is well known. I will therefore only remind you that the principles of cerebral localization rest upon the following proposition : The encephalon does not represent an homogeneous organ, a unit, but rather an association, or a confederation, composed of a certain number of diverse organs. To each of these organs belong distinct physiological properties, functions, and faculties. Now, the physiological properties of each one of these parts being known, it becomes possible to deduce therefrom the conditions of a pathological state ; this being of course but a greater or less modification of the normal state, and not a result of the intervention of new laws.

We will employ the varied knowledge furnished by normal anatomy and experimental physiology, together with those clinical observations which have been rendered reliable by a methodical and minute examination of organic lesions, and thus endeavor to ascertain upon what foundation this proposition rests. The importance and the decisive results which depend upon these last-named examinations cannot be overstated. For although normal anatomy and experimental physiology may often suggest the true direction towards localization, still nothing but the actual examination of organic lesions will permit a final decision and *furnish the proof*, at least so far as concerns the special subject of our studies—man.

A. This brings us to an examination of the encephalon under its morphological aspect. It is understood we do not attempt a rigorous description ; I propose only to draw a general outline, a knowledge of which is indispensable to our object. To simplify a very complex situation, I will confine myself to the brain ; that is, to that mass of nervous substance composed of two hemispheres and situated at the superior extremity of what are called the *cerebral peduncles* (crura cerebri).

The two hemispheres are nearly symmetrical, and so nearly identical in their structure that whatever may be said of the one may, anatomically speaking, rigidly apply to the other. Each one is enveloped in a layer of gray substance. The central part is formed by a mass of white substance, in which are furrowed the ventricles, and where are also seen, as if locked together, the central ganglionic masses, namely, the *thalami optici* and the *corpora striata*.

A transverse section made to intersect the corpora mammillaria best demonstrates the main features of the reciprocal relations of the central parts. (Fig. 1.)

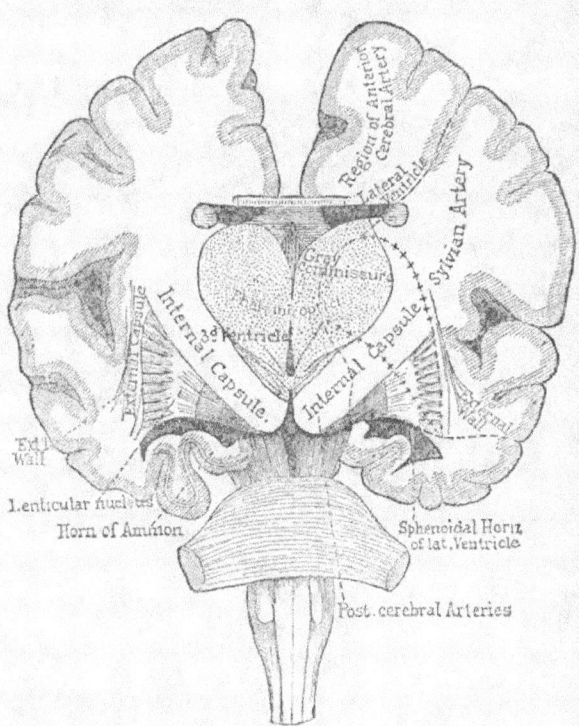

FIG. 1.—Vertico-transverse section of the brain, posterior to the tubercula mammillaria ; anterior to the peduncles.

Immediately above the protuberance you see the inferior face of the crura cerebri, the inferior portions of which issue mainly from the anterior bulbs of the pyramids.

From the lower up to the middle part of the section, you

will see two large, white tracts which run divergingly towards
the cortical portions of the hemispheres. They are between
two masses of gray substance, the one internal and superior,
the other external and inferior. These two tracts are the prolongations of the crura cerebri to the cerebral hemispheres.

The crura cerebri, which are at first irregularly quadrilateral,
become horizontally flattened as they enter the hemispheres,
running from behind forwards, and when they have passed
the narrow strait of the ganglionic region they open and
spread in every direction—in front towards the frontal extremity, in the centre towards the parietal regions, behind
towards the occipital extremity. Burdach calls the flattened
interganglionic parts of the peduncles the *internal capsules ;*
the subsequent expansion has been called by Reil the *couronne rayonnante*, diverging fibres ; the foot of the diverging fibres is where the peduncles emerge above the cerebral
ganglia. The peduncles as they enter the hemispheres somewhat resemble a *spread fan*.

Let us now describe briefly—returning to it later—the re-
spective locations of the cerebral ganglia in regard to this fan.

When, upon making the *classic section*, the lateral ventricles were opened, you will remember that there protruded
upon the surface two masses of gray substance ; the anterior
and external one is shaped like a comma or a *glass tear*, the
large extremity or head of which is anterior and the small
end or tail (cue) is posterior and lateral, and is called the
nucleus caudatus of the corpus striatum ; the other mass is
internal and posterior, and is ovoid—this is the thalamus opticus ; the thalami optici are separated by the base of the third
ventricle.

These two intraventricular gray masses, the nucleus caudatus of the corpora striata and the thalami optici, rest
above and within the peduncular fan. Below the fan, and
more voluminous than the other two, is found a third nucleus
having much the form of a plano-convex lentil, from whence
the name, *lenticulares glandulæ* (Burdach).[1] As it is of

---

[1] In French nomenclature it is called the *extra ventricular* nucleus of the
corpus striatum.

equal extent antero-posteriorly with the other two, it will always be found upon *transverse* sections (frontal sections of the Germans), perpendicular to the great interhemispheric fissure, whenever the others are met with.

The study of transverse sections, made at methodical intervals from before backward, and commenced from certain starting-points upon the base of the hemispheres, is indispensable to a familiarity with the mutual relations of the ganglia, as well as their relations to the peduncles, and it is also essential to the clinicien, whose duty is to precisely determine the parts diseased.

I will describe, as our studies may require, the appearance of these transverse sections. An understanding of one of the most posterior of these sections, made immediately in front of the crura cerebri (Fig. 1), is all that we need at the present moment.

You here see the flattened portions of the crura, the *internal capsules*. Within these are seen the surfaces of the thalami optici and the queues of the corpora striata. To the outer side of the internal capsule is seen, with its three segments, the lenticular nucleus of the corpus striatum. These gray nuclei are possibly so many centres endowed with distinct properties and functions; but it must be remembered that this is not yet positively demonstrated. Still external to the lenticular bodies you will discover, in succession, the external capsules, the outer walls (little white unnamed bands), and lastly the gray layers of the island of Reil.

I have no intention to engage at present with details of structure; I wish only to insist upon these designations given, however minute they may seem; for years past I have persisted in introducing them into the French nomenclature only because I have considered them of the highest utility when, as upon autopsy, it is desirable to indicate the exact locality of the lesion. Who would dare to affirm that such or such a region, which has no place in our nomenclature, is not possessed of an importance even of the first order? Besides, how can such region be described in a record of autopsy if it has no recognized name? The names which I supply furnish many starting-points, and their utility is therefore incontestable. Is a good strategic chart ever too complete? It is in thus precisely specifying the spot occupied by a hemorrhagic centre—the external or internal capsules, the gray ganglia, the foot of the diverging fibres, etc.— that you will be able to prove whether there are symptomatic differences of location such as might aid prognosis. An example, presented in a case of cerebral hæmorrhage, will serve as proof that this is no superfluous labor. If a hæmorrhagic centre involves only the external capsule, whatever be the extent of the lesion, the patient in all probability will recover without persistence of hemiplegia or any other infirmity; but, on the contrary, if it be the internal capsule that is involved, and the patient survives, there will remain persistent paralysis and permanent contractions.

The importance of an exact and minute study of the shape and plan of the brain, joined to an appropriate nomenclature, is especially shown when dealing with the *convolutions* upon the surface of hemispheres. For a long time these convolutions were supposed to be, as it were, the result of chance, and thus they escaped any close description. Leuret and Gratiolet demonstrated that, on the contrary, there was an orderly plan, which could be traced from the inferior mammalia, by the way of the monkey, up to man.

Moreover, there are among the convolutions those which can be called *fundamental*, for the reason that their locations and relations are absolutely fixed; then again there are those which may be termed *secondary*, or accessory, and which must be studied abstractly, because they are *variable*.

You will easily comprehend that without a good topography of the convolutions it is quite impossible to take one step in the more important knowledge of cerebral localizations. For example, how can we speak of lesions producing aphasia unless we are able to determine precisely the location and form of the third frontal convolution? How could we locate in man the regions called psycho-motor, which the studies of Fritsch, Hitzig, and Ferrier have discovered in animals, if no notice be taken of the convolutions and

furrows upon the gray substance of the parietal lobes and the
posterior portions of the frontal lobes? How many observations which might have thrown light upon these interesting
questions of localization are valueless, for the reason that,
from an insufficient knowledge of the altered parts, an exact
description has not been possible! In order to obviate as
far as possible that lack in the anatomical description of the
normal brain, I have for a long time past habituated myself
to outlining the locations of brain-lesions upon schemes designed from nature. In the absence of these precautions
no ideas can be obtained which are not open to criticism.
Still, this study has not so many difficulties as may at first be
supposed. If the most complete knowledge has not yet found
its way into classic works, it nevertheless abounds elsewhere.
Beyond the standard works of Leuret and Gratiolet, Bishoff,
Arnold, Turner, etc. (a familiarity with which is indispensable), I recommend to your use the little manual of Ecker,[1]
which contains good topographical plates, accompanied with
a simple nomenclature, together with synonyms. Through
my advice Duret has employed these plates in his important
mémoire upon the circulation in the encephalon. An excel-
lent work upon this subject, also, is a thesis by Gromier, written
under the inspiration of Paul Broca, and entitled, "*Study
upon Cerebral Convolutions in Man and Monkey.* 1874."

Comparative anatomy is also a powerful adjunct in the
study of the convolutions. Between the monkey and man,
for example, the resemblance is striking,[2] as concerns the fundamental convolutions and furrows, and that arrangement,
which in man is somewhat unintelligible, is explained in the
brain of the monkey by reason of its greater simplicity. I
therefore will exhibit a sketch of the convolutions as observed in the monkey before considering those of the human

[1] *Die Hirnwindungen des Menschen nach eigenen Untersuchungen insbesondere
über die Entwicklung derselben beim Fötus und mit Rücksicht auf das Bedürf-
niss der Ärzte.* Brunswick, 1869. There is an English translation of the work.

[2] Upon this subject, read in the last edition of Darwin's "The Descent of
Man" (London, 1874), Professor Huxley's interesting note (p. 199), on the resem-
blances and differences in the structure and development of the brain in man and
apes.

brain. This study possesses additional interest from the fact that actual experiment has already located upon some of the convolutions of the monkey brain those points known as *psychomotor*, thus furnishing a base for clinical and anatomico-pathological research concerning their existence in corresponding points of the human brain.

Here is a lateral representation of a monkey's brain (Fig. 2)

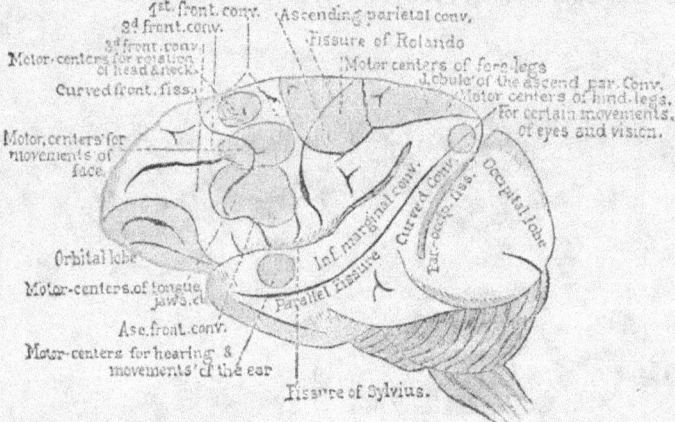

FIG. 2.—External face of the brain of the magot monkey (Pithecus Innuus). —*Broca and Gromier.*

taken from the work of Gromier. It is a brain of the magot (*Pithecus innuus*), a monkey of somewhat low type. I will give a description of the external face of the hemisphere only, the internal and inferior faces being of less importance to our subject.

First, two long fissures are seen, the fissure of Rolando and that of Sylvius. These fissures converge and constitute the posterior border of the external face of the frontal lobe.

Further back is seen another fissure, the *parieto-occipital.* In the monkey this fissure very clearly separates the occipital lobe from the temporal and parietal lobes. This separation is much less marked in the human brain on account of the overlying convolutions (*plis de passage*) which more or less conceal it.

The parietal and sphenoidal lobes are less distinguishable in the monkey, and to complete the outline it is necessary to prolong the fissure of Sylvius with an imaginary line passing a convolution called the *gyrus angularis* (*pli courbe.*)

The external surface of the cerebral hemisphere is divided into four lobes, the frontal, parietal, sphenoidal, and occipital.

Each of these lobes is subdivided by fissures or sulci of the second order into secondary lobes, called convolutions.

Frontal Lobes.— *The præcentral or curved frontal fissure* in the frontal lobe is the anterior border of a convolution lying parallel with the fissures of Sylvius called the *ascending frontal convolution*, and to give it more interest, I will observe that in its superior extremity Ferrier locates the motor centres of the opposite upper limbs.

Fissures running at right angles with the *curved frontal fissure* divide the remainder of the frontal lobe into three convolutions. 1st. In the posterior extremity of the first or upper convolution Ferrier places the motor centre for the movement of the head; 2d. Upon the same authority the posterior part of the second or middle convolution is the centre of facial movements; 3d. In the third or lower convolution is located, in the monkey, a motor centre for movements of the lips and tongue; to this part is ascribed in man the faculty of articulate speech—the third convolution, or as the English call it, *Broca's convolution*. I do not wish to be less French than are the English, and in adopting the term I am happy to recognize the signal service which our colleague has rendered to the cause of cerebral localization.

Parietal Lobe.—The parietal lobe, so difficult of study in man, is on the contrary very easy in the monkey. The interparietal fissure divides it into two secondary lobes : 1st. The *superior parietal lobe*, where Ferrier locates the centre for movements of the lower limbs; 2d. The *inferior parietal lobe;* 3d. A fissure, more marked in the higher monkeys, separates the parietal lobes from the ascending parietal convolution. In a part of the ascending parietal convolution, and extending to the superior extremity of the ascending frontal convolution, is the motor centre of the upper limbs.

Sphenoidal Lobe.—The situation of the sphenoidal lobe is easily understood. Upon the convex face of the hemisphere it is bounded by the lower border of the hemisphere and by the fissure of Sylvius. The *parallel fissure,* called thus because it is parallel to the fissure of Sylvius, divides the lobe into two parts. In the upper part is found the marginal convolution, and at the posterior end of the fissure, the gyrus angularis, the removal of which Ferrier says produces temporary blindness of the opposite eye.

Occipital Lobe.—A transverse furrow separates this lobe into two parts. For the present there is nothing special to be said of it.

After this brief survey of the cerebral convolutions in the monkey, the corresponding ones in man become more sim-

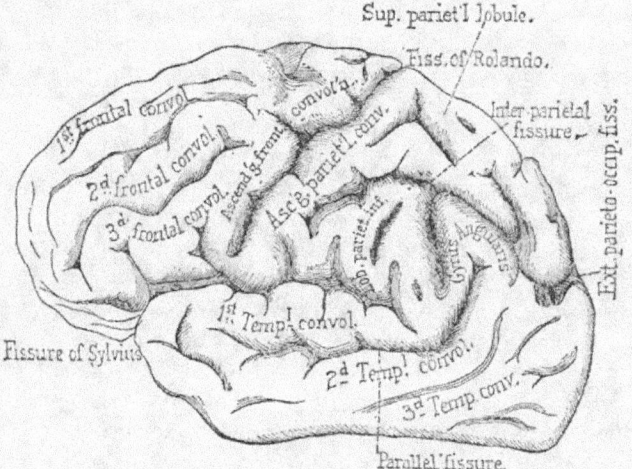

FIG. 3.—Convex surface of a hemisphere of the human brain (parietal lobe partly schematic.)

plified, as proved by the recapitulation which I will now give, using for that purpose a plate from Foville's beautiful work (Fig. 3).

You observe that the fissure of Sylvius and the fissure of Rolando furnish the inferior and posterior borders of the frontal lobe, in which lobe you may notice the ascending frontal (or anterior parietal) convolution and the first, second and third frontal convolutions. (Fig. 3.)

The parieto-occipital fissure, on account of its overlying folds (*plis de passage*), affords but a confused separation between the occipital, parietal, and sphenoidal lobes.

Back of the fissure of Rolando, between that and the interparietal fissure, is the ascending parietal convolution ; above and back of the interparietal fissure you will find, successively, the superior and inferior parietal lobules and the gyrus angularis.

In the sphenoidal or temporal lobe, the brain, both of the human and the monkey, has a fissure that extends to the gyrus angularis ; this is the parallel fissure ; between it and the fissure of Sylvius lies the first temporal convolution ; below and posterior are the two other temporal convolutions.

The parietal lobe, the fissure of Sylvius and that of Rolando, afford a sufficient number of starting-points to serve as guides in autopsy.

III.—Thus the surface of the brain is marked off into divisions, the invariableness of which cannot be misunderstood. Do these various fundamental convolutions represent distinct functional centres ? A consideration of only the external achitecture cannot resolve the question.

We will now resort to the microscope to ascertain whether a comparative study of structure in the various regions of the cortex will not furnish still more significant information upon this subject.

Unaided vision has long since recognized differences of structure in the gray substance, according to the encephalic region examined. From this point of view let us examine, for example, the lower portion of the occipital lobe. In those parts of the lobe which surround the posterior cornua of the lateral ventricles, the gray substance is not of that almost uniform appearance which belongs to other regions of the brain, as, for instance, to the anterior lobes. Vicq d'Azyr observed that in those parts of the occipital lobes the gray substance of the convolutions was very clearly divided into two secondary bands, separated by a white line which is still called the *band of Vicq d'Azyr*.   In this respect also the unassisted eye can distinguish between the gray substance of the cornua Ammonis, the isle of Reil, and that of other regions of the hemispheres.

To appreciate the value of these facts it is necessary to enter more into detail.

SECOND LECTURE.

STRUCTURE OF THE GRAY SUBSTANCE OF THE BRAIN.

*Summary :—*General Structural Character of the Brain-Cortex.—1st ; Ganglionic or Nerve Cells ; Pyramidal Cells.—Views Respecting the Nerve-Cells of the Anterior Cornua of the Gray Substance of the Spinal Cord (Motor-Cells) ; Size, Form, Body, Nucleus, Nucleolus, Protoplasma, Fibrillæ and Granules ; Nerve Network ; Prolongations of Protoplasma ; Nerve-Prolongations.—Comparison of the Motor Nerve-Cells of the Spinal Cord with the Pyramidal Cells.—Pyramidal Cells ; Size ; the Small Cells ; the Large or Giant Cells ; Composition of the Cells ; Shape, Body, Nucleus, Nucleolus ; Cellular Prolongations ; Pyramidal Prolongations ; Prolongations which Recall those of the Protoplasma ; Basal Prolongations.—2d and 3d ; Elements of Globular Cells ; Elongated Cells.—4th and 5th ; Medullary Tubes ; Neuroglia or Amorphous Cerebral Substance.—Relations between the Elements ; Five-layer Type.—The Importance of Examining the Gray Substance of each Convolution.—Two Divisions, Structurally, of the Gray Substance.—Labors of Betz.

GENTLEMEN :

I. The structure of the gray substance, in whatever region of the hemispheres, presents certain general characteristics which should be examined before approaching distinctive characteristics. All parts of the cortex are composed of essentially the same elements. Each one of the composing elements may present important relative deviations from the standard type, according to the region observed ; and in a *regional study* of the gray substance great weight should be given to the different proportion and manner in which these elements are distributed in different parts.

After having examined these components individually, we will investigate as to how they combine to form the gray substance. Our description will commence with those elements which play the principal rôle, that is, those *ganglionic* or *nerve-cells* which are the special characteristic elements of this region ; they are usually called the *pyramidal cells*.

In order to fully appreciate the morphological properties of these elements, perhaps it is best not to confine our attention to them exclusively. I have thought best to employ the comparative method, reposing upon the common saying : "Light is born from contrast" (" *La lumière naît du contraste* ").

I will first recite the principal traits of that nerve cellular element which is at present best understood : I refer to the *nerve-cells of the anterior cornua of the gray substance of the spinal cord*, called the *motor cells*. The abridged description which I will give of these nerve-cells will serve as a type. In the comparisons that follow I shall point out more than one difference, but I shall also make special mention of more than one remarkable analogy.

The *motor cells* are cells without a distinct membrane, the *diameters* of which are variable, though not deviating greatly from 0.050 m. Gerlach, however, says that they may reach to 0.120 m. Their *form* is more or less globular, rarely elongated. The bodies are composed of protoplasm which appears granular when seen in the non-living state, but in the serum, or after the action of osmic acid upon the fresh cell, it appears to be composed of a transparent protoplasm in the interior of which, as Shultz has demonstrated, exist numerous *fibrillæ*. These fibrillæ by post-mortem alterations change to granules. The cell contains a nucleus and a brilliant nucleolus. I also generally observe in the protoplasm, even in its physiological condition, the presence of brown *pigmentary granules*.

One of the most important peculiarities of these cells, however, is that they are armed with numerous prolongations, which have a voluminous trunk as they leave the cells, and which become smaller in proportion as they extend and divide (dichotomously). The last of these ramifications are extremely minute, and it is difficult to trace them for any distance.

Gerlach, after the use of preparations of chloride of gold,

asserts that these ramifications terminate in a sort of anastomosing network which he called *réseau nerveux*. These prolongations are composed, like the cell-bodies themselves, of granular protoplasm and long parallel filaments, which may be traced into the body of the cells. They are called *protoplasmic prolongations*, in order to distinguish them from another species of prolongation which I will now describe.

A German histologist, Deiters, some years ago discovered an important fact which has since been verified by all anatomists. It is that the greater part, if not all, of the motor cells possess, besides the prolongation which we have described, a prolongation (one only for each cell) which characteristically differs from the others. These prolongations bear the name of *nerve-prolongations*, and the reason of that qualification will be presently understood. It proceeds from the body of the cell, or from one of its larger prolongations, in the form of a very slender filament, but which, little by little, becomes more voluminous. This prolongation does not ramify, and it becomes less brightly colored by action of carmine than do the *protoplasmic prolongations*.

If followed a sufficient distance, it is found to be enveloped, the same as an ordinary nerve, with a myeline cylinder, so that it may be considered as a cylinder axis at its origin, and at a certain distance as a complete nerve. The connection of the nerve-cells with the tubes of the medullary substance, by means of these prolongations (nerves), is then beyond doubt.

Such are the principal characters of the spinal motor nerve-cells; and here seems the place to observe the characteristics of the *pyramidal cells of the gray cortex* (Fig. 4).

These cells are quite variable in dimensions, the most of them are relatively very small. The pyramidal cells, which may be placed in this class, have at the base a mean diameter of 0.010 m. Those of the larger sort, less in number than the preceding, generally occupy the lower portion of the layer of pyramidal cells. Their diameter attains to 0.022 m. (Koschewnikoff).

Finally there are giant pyramidal cells (Riesenzellen).

They have been carefully studied by Betz (of Kiew) and by Mierzejewski. They are found in certain well-determined regions of the gray cortex. The diameters of these gigantic cells sometimes reach 0.040 m. to 0.050 m., that is, they equal the cells of the anterior cornua of the spinal cord.

However they may differ in dimensions, the essential structure of the pyramidal cells appears always the same. Therefore, for convenience' sake, we will study the larger kind, or the *giant-cells*.

To a certain point the term *pyramidal cells* may be used literally; their form resembles, indeed, a more or less elongated pyramid. The *body* of the cell recalls the description which we have just given, and Schultz records that he has seen fibre-like structure in it. The *nucleus*, according to very many authors, is angular, and reproduces in a certain degree the general form of the cell. The *nucleolus* itself presents nothing special.

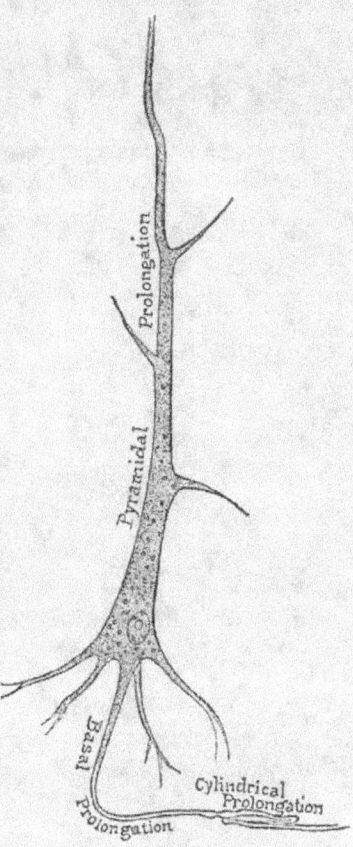

FIG. 4.—Pyramidal prolongation.

The cellular prolongations offer peculiarities worthy of interest. One of them may be called *pyramidal prolongations*, for it is, as it were, the body of the cell progressively narrowed. As they extend they give off lateral branches, and at their extremities they often divide in form of a fork, and

2

this extremity is always directed towards the surface of the convolution. It follows that the cell is situated so that its base is parallel to the interior or medullary border of the zone of the gray cortex.

Other prolongations of the same category extend sometimes from the angles, sometimes from the base, and they ramify in such manner as to recall the protoplasmic prolongations of the spinal motor cells. Do these prolongations terminate in a nerve network in the gray cortex, the same as Gerlach says occurs with the spinal cells? Some authors say they do.

There certainly exist for the larger pyramidal cells, for the giant-cells, and perhaps for the small cells, cylindrical prolongations quite analogous to those of the spinal motor cells. In both, the origin is a slender filament which soon becomes somewhat larger. Upon successful dissections it is possible, at a certain distance from the cell, to discover that the prolongations are covered with a cylinder of myeline. Koschewnikoff[1] placed this fact beyond doubt by examination of cells from the anterior lobes of the brain of one who died from encephalitis; and since the publication of his work the reality of his description has often been demonstrated by others. These *basilar prolongations*, to use Meynert's expression, are always turned towards the medullary substance of the convolutions.

That which we have adduced makes it impossible to misunderstand the analogies associating the pyramidal cells of the gray cortex—at least the large cells and the giant-cells—with the motor cells of the anterior cornua of the spinal cord; and these analogies (already described by Luys: J. Luys, *Recherches sur le système nerveux, etc.*, p. 162 et suiv., Paris, 1865) we must consider later.

---

[1] A. Koschewnikoff.—Axencylinderforsätz der Nervenzellen im kleinen Hirn des Kalbes. In Schultze's Archiv, p. 332, 1869. Axencylinderforsätz der Nervenzellen aus der Grosshirnrinde. Idem, 1869. p. 375. Betz, Centralblatt, 1874. p. 579; Mierzejewski, Études sur les lésions cérébrales dans la paralysie générale, in Archives de physiologie, p. 194, 1875. J. Batty Tuke, Morisonian Lectures, in Edinb. Med. Journal, p. 394, May, 1874.

The pyramidal cells are not the only elements found in the gray substance. There are also small globular cells (rarely pyramidal), measuring from 0.008 m. to 0.010 m. (Meynert),[1] sometimes furnished with small prolongations; they are generally sparse, though sometimes, or at some points, they form a tolerably thick layer. Various writers have regarded them as incompletely developed nerve-elements; others again have denied them this character, and compare them to the elements which constitute the granular layer of the retina.

Meynert ranks also among the nerve-elements of the cortical zones a kind of elongated, generally fusiform, ramified cell, and which at certain points constitutes a fifth layer. These cells generally have their grand axis directed parallel with the fibres which connect the convolutions (*the system of association*), medullary fibres that run from one convolution to another (fibræ arcuatæ); the last-named cells seem to make a part of that system.

These, then, are the cellular nerve-elements, so reputed, which enter into the structure of the gray substance. Besides these, there are other elements which we ought to mention: the *medullary tubes* and the *amorphous cerebral substance* (neuroglia). To these last, which penetrate the gray substance as fasciculi, we will return later. As for the neuroglia, still known under the name of *formation épendymaire* (Rokitansky), that serves as an amorphous uniting substance. I will not enter into the detail of the peculiarities of structure relative to the neuroglia of the gray substance. I will only remark that latterly it has been considered by various authors as composed of a peculiar kind of conjunctive cells, the bodies of which contain very little protoplasm, and are furnished with non-ramified prolongations (*cellules araignées de Boll et Golgi*). These prolongations, entangled and cemented by an interposed gelatinous substance, would be considered as composing the entire mass of neuroglia. We must examine that interpretation. Without denying the normal existence, in certain regions, of ramifying cells (*cellules de Deiters*), I will

---

[1] Meynert.—Stricker's Handb., t. II., et traduct. anglaise, t. II., p. 381 et suiv.

remark that the gray substance in that respect is very likely fashioned upon the same model as is the white. In other words, the neuroglia resembles the type of ordinary conjunctive tissue, conjunctive fasciculi, and flat cells (Ranvier) ; only in the neuroglia the fibrous filaments would be freer than elsewhere. For the present, I omit the study of the vessels ; they will shortly receive our special attention.

This suffices, I think, concerning the individual history of the various elements which compose the gray substance. We should now examine the method in which these elements are arranged, in order to see what may be the difference in arrangement, as well also as in respect to the constitution of the elements themselves, in each of the various regions which are divided off by the main fissures on the surface of the brain.

There is a certain arrangement which may be considered as representing the most common type, and it is also the most widely extended ; it is the one that in thin slices may be distinguished with the microscope, and which presents five successive layers. It is met with nearly everywhere in the anterior lobes. The elements are separated as follows :

1. The *first layer*, the one nearest the meninges, is composed almost exclusively of conjunctive substance. There the nerve-elements are very scarce ; Kölliker and Arndt,[1] however, describe a layer near the surface, under the pia mater, of very delicate parallel nerve-tubes. The nerve-cells in this locality are very sparse. To the naked eye that layer has the appearance of a little white zone. The absence of color seems due to the poverty of nerve-elements and to the small number of capillary vessels contained in the layer. Indeed the arterioles penetrating the cortex do not furnish numerous capillaries except to the lower layer. That peculiarity of structure is very well indicated in a plate by Henle,[2] and in a cut in the *mémoire* of Duret.[3]

[1] R. Arndt.—Studien über die Architektonick der Grosshirnrinde des Menschen, in Arch. für mikroskop. Anatomie, 3d Bd.—1867, p. 441, Taf. xxiii., Fig. 1, a, et Fig. 2.

[2] J. Henle.—Handb. der Nervenlehre, p. 274, Fig. 201, Braunschweig, 1871.

[3] Archives de Physiologie, T. vi., pl. 6, Figs. 2 et 3.

2. The second layer (Fig. 5) is marked by an agglomeration of pyramidal nerve-cells of the small species,[1] numerous and very close together, which give it a decided gray color.

3. The third layer (Fig. 5) is chiefly composed of pyramidal cells, some of the medium size and some voluminous. The latter, more separated from each other than the first, are generally situated at the lower part of the layer, and penetrate even into the next (fourth) layer. Besides the cells there are to be found in the third layer fasciculi of medullary fibres which dip perpendicularly to the surface of the cortex, forming as it were columns between the groups of pyramidal cells. This arrangement has been faithfully represented by Luys[1] and by Henle.[2] It is in the lower portions of the third layer that in some regions the giant-cells exist. It would seem as though the rarity of cells and the presence of medullary fibres ought to give this layer a white appearance; it really has a yellowish color, prob-

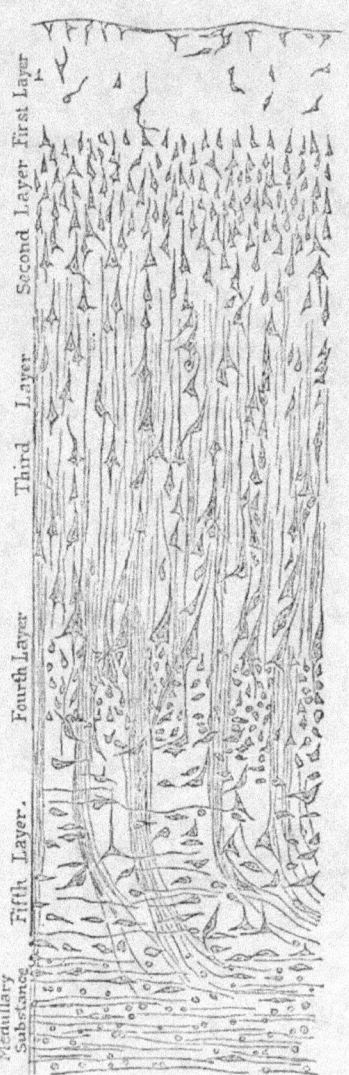

FIG. 5.—Five-layer type of cerebral cortex. (Brain of mammalia.) — *Meynert. From Stricker's Hand-book.* T. II., p. 704.

[1] Atlas, etc., pl. xx., Fig. 4.

[2] Loc. cit., Fig. 198, p. 271.

ably from the presence of pigment and the abundance of capillary vessels.

4. Then comes the *fourth layer* (Fig. 5), where are seen the globular cells with ill-determined characters, and the *fifth layer*, where are found the fusiform cells of which we have just spoken.

These summary investigations have enabled us to appreciate the interest which might result from an examination of the structure of the gray cortical substance, made convolution by convolution. It has long been known that the different regions of the gray cortex differ notably from each other in point of structure. But the most recent and fertile study in this direction is by Betz, the results of which have been published in the Centralblatt of the past year.[1] Betz proposes examining the modifications of texture of the gray substance, convolution by convolution. In this respect he claims that on the surfaces of the hemispheres there are two fundamental regions which are nearly divided by the fissure of Rolando.

Anterior to that furrow the gray cortex is characterized by a predominance of large pyramidal cells over the globular cells. The orbital region is included in this division.

Back of the furrow this region embraces all the sphenoidal and occipital lobes and the median portion, to the anterior border of the quadrilateral lobule. There the granular cells preponderate, and the large ones are relatively rare.

Besides this there is a special department in each of these regions which deserves attention. We will deal first with that of the posterior region.

1st. Here, the well-developed nerve-elements are the tolerably large cells. According to Meynert they were the largest found in the cortex of the hemispheres before the discovery of the giant-cells. They are sometimes the 0.030 m. in diameter. The protoplasmic prolongations are not numerous ; the basilar prolongations are directed horizontally, and sometimes constitute communications between the cells.

---

[1] P. Betz, of Kiew.—Anatomischer Nachweis Zweier Gehirncentra. In Centralblatt, 1874, Nos. 37 et 38.

The territory where that character is observed includes (*a*) the *cuneus*; (*b*) the posterior half of the lingual and fusiform lobules ; (*c*) all the occipital lobe ; (*d*) the first two sphenoidal convolutions and the transition convolution (*pli de passage*). According to Betz, this region is devoted to the functions of sensibility. From other reasons of an anatomical order, to which we will revert, the posterior parts of the brain have for a long time past been spoken of as the seat of the sensorium.

2d. The anterior lobe deserves particular notice, and may be called (you will see why) the department of the *giant pyramidal cells*, or the *motor cells par excellence*. This department embraces the entire ascending frontal convolution, the superior extremity of the ascending parietal convolution, together with a part which we will soon study under the name of *paracentral lobule*, and which is situated upon the internal face of the hemisphere at the extremity of the ascending convolutions. It is here that exist almost exclusively the giant-cells. Their distribution is not uniform, for they are more numerous than elsewhere at the superior extremity of the two middle convolutions, and above all in the paracentral lobule. They are located in groups or islands. They are to be found in certain points, which will be indicated, in all species of monkeys, the inferior as well as the chimpanzee. Indeed Betz has observed in the dog the same kind of cells at those points designated by Fritsch and Hitzig as motor centres—otherwise spoken of as the parts neighboring the *sulcus cruciatus*. Interest is added by the fact that in the dog the giant pyramidal cells exist nowhere else but in the regions called psycho-motor. It doubtless has not escaped your notice that in the monkey the distribution of the large nerve-cells very closely corresponds to those convolutions where experiments, in the hands of Ferrier, have demonstrated the existence of motor points, namely, in the central convolutions. This is an interesting result furnished by histological study, and which, combined with experimental or anatomico-pathological results, cannot fail to throw some light upon the development of cerebral localizations.

THIRD LECTURE.

CONSIDERATIONS UPON THE NORMAL STRUCTURE OF THE GRAY SUBSTANCE OF THE CONVOLUTIONS.

(CONTINUATION.)

Summary:—Description of a Section of the Gray Matter of the Cerebellum.—Type of the Five-Layer Stratifications of Cellular Nerve-Elements.—Regions where this Type of Stratification Exists.—Department of Pyramidal or Giant-Cells.—Relations between the Cells and the Psycho-motor Centres.—Description of the Internal Face of the Cerebral Hemispheres.—Paracentral Lobule.—Ascending Convolutions.—Clinical and Experimental Facts Relative to the Development of the Pyramidal Giant-Cells.—Structure of the Gray Matter in the Posterior Regions of the Encephalon.

GENTLEMEN :

Before proceeding further towards the purpose of our subject—the theory of localization in cerebral maladies—I ought to complete the matter broached in the last lecture, relative to the differences in the normal structure of the gray matter, as found in the various convolutions of the cerebral hemispheres.

A. We will first examine the common type, or the one most generally and best understood. With Meynert, one may call it the *five-layer type of cellular nerve-elements—so reputed*.

I will briefly recall the characteristic traits of that type. To assist in this let us again glance at Fig. 5, a section of the third frontal convolution at the base of a fissure.

As a contrast, we will run over the description of a section of the gray substance of the cerebellum ; this description, like the preceding one, is borrowed from Meynert. In the gray substance of the cerebellum there are, in successive order : 1st. A thick layer, poor in cellular elements, and which receives the protoplasmic prolongations from the nerve-cells of the subjacent layer.   2d. Below this, a layer where are found, according to Meynert, fusiform cells and medullary fibres running parallel to the line of limit.   3d. Still lower, the cells of Purkinje, which occupy the superior portion of a very granular layer ; below all, the medullary substance.[1]

If you now examine the figure representing the five layers of gray substance of the brain proper (cerebrum), you will see that the gray substance is not fashioned in all parts of the encephalon upon the same model.   I shall shortly show you the very well-defined though not so strongly marked differences that are apparent according to the different regions examined in the cerebrum ; but first I must return to the five-layer type.

B. The arrangement thus designated exists in all the brain anterior to the fissure of Rolando, as well also as a little back of it, in a portion of the parietal lobes which is indistinctly separated from the border of the occipital lobe.   We will presently see that this type is notably modified in the posterior part of the encephalon, including, 1st. All the sphenoidal lobe ; 2d. The occipital lobe ; and 3d. The gray matter of that portion of the internal face which is circumscribed by the posterior extremity of the occipital lobe and by a furrow which is the posterior limit of a distinct region, which we will shortly describe under the name of the quadrilateral lobule.

(*a.*) For greater clearness it is necessary to revisit a point already surveyed ; namely, that in those regions of the hemispheres occupied exclusively by the five-layer type, there exists a department of itself, where the gray structure is distinguished by an interesting peculiarity ; which is, the invariable presence in those parts of comparatively enormous pyramidal cells, and which, on account of their size, are called *giant-cells.*   While these cells retain the pyramidal form common to the cellular nerve-elements of these regions, they differ not only in dimensions, but also by the distinctness of their nerve-prolongations and by the development of their proto-

---

[1] Voir aussi Henle, Nervenlehre, etc., Figs. 162, 163 A, 163 B.

plasmic prolongations. This last trait permits their comparison with the motor nerve-cells of the anterior cornua of the spinal cord.

The regions of this important peculiarity are the central regions of the external surface of the hemisphere, to wit: the *ascending frontal convolution, the ascending parietal convolution*, especially at their superior parts, and finally in a little lobule situated upon the internal face of the hemisphere, until recently unnamed, and which Betz has proposed to call the *paracentral lobule*. (Fig. 6.)

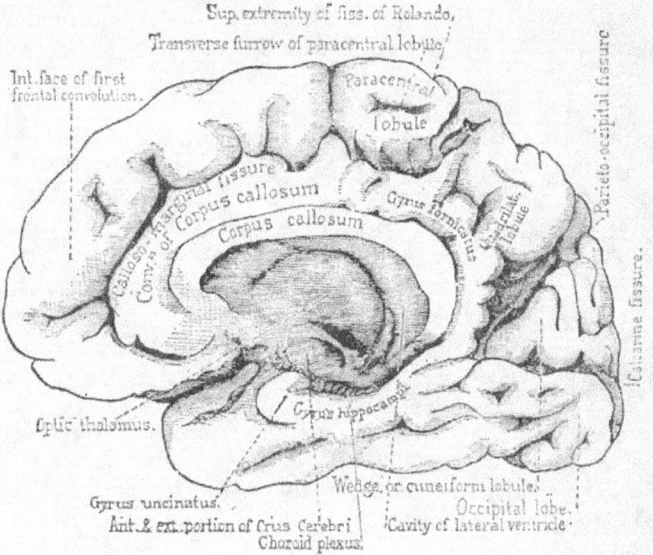

FIG. 6.—Internal surface of right hemisphere of a human brain. (*Drawn from nature.*)[1]

I would remind you that the existence of the giant-cells in the gray matter, and their localization in the regions above indicated, were discovered by Betz and Mierzejewski. The results obtained by these authors have recently been con-

---

[1] Respecting the topography of the median face of the cerebrum, consult pl. viii. of Foville's Atlas, and Fig. 4 of Ecker's work.

firmed by J. Batty Tuke in his lectures at Edinburgh.[1] I have myself also verified the same.

I again remind you that the regions remarkable for this peculiarity of structure are precisely those where, in the monkey, according to Ferrier,[2] the psycho-motor centres of the limbs are located. Is not that a coincidence worthy of your attention? Let us recall the fact also that, in the dog, those parts reputed, through the experiments of Ferrier and by the previous ones of Hitzig, as excito-motor, are said by Betz to be distinguished by the presence of giant pyramidal cells—cells which in these animals are to be found in no other part of the gray matter. I think my persistence justified by the necessity of fixing in your minds as exactly as possible all these details.

(b.) These facts give a very special interest to those regions of the hemispheres which possess this anatomical peculiarity. I therefore feel that a thorough topographic knowledge of those regions is of the utmost use in order to be able to indicate them with precision in the records of autopsies, and consequently I will enter this subject more fully. In so doing we shall of course have occasion to describe the configuration of the middle faces of the hemispheres, a region which up to the present time, in my opinion, has remained too little known.

The arrangement of the ascending convolutions, their origin at the superior border of the hemispheres, are now so familiar to us that our attention can be turned to the arrangement of the internal or median faces of the hemispheres. In that section (Fig. 6) which divides the corpus callosum anteroposteriorly you first see at the centre the divided surface of the grand commissure; below, the *septum lucidum*, the internal face of the thalamus opticus, then the cut surfaces of the crura cerebri.

Better to obtain our points of compass, we will start from a

---

[1] Edinburgh Med. Jour., Nov., 1874, p. 394.

[2] West Riding Asylum, t. IV., pp. 49 and 50, Proceedings of the Royal Society, No. 151, 1874. British Medical Journal, Dec. 19, 1874.

familiar landmark upon the external face of the brain, that is, the fissure of Rolando, and follow it to its extreme internal end. This furrow sometimes stops a little short of the inter-hemispheric fissure; at other times it extends quite to it, making a sort of notch on its superior border.

The paracentral lobule is located immediately below that point. It is bounded as follows : *posteriorly*, by an oblique fissure, which is the posterior prolongation of the calloso-marginal (that fissure extended constitutes the posterior border of the ascending parietal convolution) ; *below*, by that horizontal portion of the calloso-marginal fissure which separates it from the convolution of the corpus callosum (called *gyrus fornicatus*) ; *anteriorly*, by a fissure generally shallow, but which sometimes continues upon the internal face of the hemispheres and which anteriorly marks the internal part of the ascending frontal convolution and bounds the anterior face of the paracentral lobule.

Thus we have a small quadrilateral lobule whose greatest diameter is antero-posterior. Generally a shallow furrow, midway between the upper and lower borders, runs the entire length of the lobule. By reason of its structure, as much as from its position, it may be said that the paracentral lobule seems to represent upon the median face of the hemisphere the inverse surfaces, the internal extremities of the two ascending convolutions.

This point fixed, it is not difficult to give the remaining topography of the internal face of the hemispheres. 1st. Anterior to the paracentral lobule is seen the median surface of the first frontal convolution. 2d. Below, and separated from the preceding by the calloso-marginal furrow, is the convolution of the corpus callosum (*gyrus fornicatus*). 3d. The last-named convolution is continued posteriorly, forming a lobule quite circumscribed, and which is called the quadrilateral lobule (*avant coin, Vorzwickel, præcuncus*). This lobule we may consider as the internal or median face of the superior parietal lobule. Behind this the *temporo-occipital fissure* (very marked at this point, because it is not interrupted, as upon its external face, by overlying convolutions) separates very clearly the quadrilateral lobule from the occipital lobe. 4th. Immediately behind the quadrilateral lobule in the region of the occipital lobe, there is a triangular lobule, the point of which is inferio-anterior, the base posterio-superior, and which is bounded posteriorly by a deep fissure, the *fissura calcarina*; that little lobule is called the *cuneus* (*coin*, *zwickel*). 5th. Below that triangle you observe the lack of demarcation already noticed upon the external surface between the occipito-sphenoidal lobes. In this region should be specially observed two convolutions running antero-posteriorly. They are : (*a*) the lateral occipito-sphenoidal lobule (*lobulus fusiformis*); (*b*) the median occipito-sphenoidal lobule (*lobulus lingualis*). 6th. Still in front, and fully within the sphenoidal lobe, is the *gyrus hippocampi*, the hook (*crochet*) which constitutes part of the *horn of Ammon* (*cornu Ammonis*).

As we proceed we shall most certainly have occasion to use the topographical knowledge which we are obtaining, and I hasten to complete the description, which in some respects is a digression.

C. I therefore return to the *paracentral lobule* and to the *ascending convolutions*. These have already a history in experimental pathology, and further on it will be shown that they have also a history in human pathology. I am not aware whether with the monkey, at least with the higher grade of monkey, the paracentral lobule (which exists as with man) has ever been the object of physiological investigations.

(*a.*) I may here cite a case, unique of its kind to be sure, but which nevertheless will for the future lend an interest to this lobule as connected with human pathology. This instance, of which I give an outline, has been recorded by an attentive observer, Sander.[1]

A child who died at the age of fifteen had been attacked in the third year of its age with *infantile spinal paralysis*. The malady had included and more or less atrophied all the limbs, and especially those of the left side. Autopsy revealed in

---

[1] Centralblatt, 1875.

the spinal cord all the lesions described by the French authors. A minute examination of the brain led to the discovery that the two ascending convolutions upon the external face were very much shorter than normal. They left the island of Reil somewhat uncovered, besides which they were destitute of folds. The paracentral lobule was entirely rudimentary, in this respect markedly in contrast with all the other convolutions, which were perfectly developed. Lastly, the lesions were most pronounced in the right hemisphere, which is in keeping with the circumstance that the spinal lesions were most marked upon the left side.

The author expresses the opinion that in this case the limbs having, at an early age, suffered complete paralysis, resulting from a profound spinal lesion, the psycho-motor centres, struck with inertia at a time when they were in process of evolution, had in consequence been arrested in development. The interpretation seems worthy of consideration. It is much to be regretted that the condition of the nerve-cells in the psycho-motor centres was not ascertained.

A case observed by Luys to a certain extent resembles the foregoing. In a subject where amputation had been made, some years previous to autopsy, my colleague at *la Salpê-trière* noted an atrophy of the cerebral convolution on the side opposite to the amputation. Unfortunately the exact seat of the atrophy was not (to my knowledge, at least) given.

(*b.*) I am thus led to introduce another fact concerning that part of the brain with which we are occupied. According to the researches of Betz, the giant pyramidal cells exist but in small number with very young infants; it is only later that their number increases, and that increase is effected, according to all appearances, under the influence of functional exercise.

This fact is worthy of being joined, on the one hand, with that of Sander's, and on the other hand to an observation of an experimental order recently recorded by Soltmann.[1] That author (and I believe that Professor Rouget, of Montpellier,

---

[1] Reizbarkeit der Grosshirnrinde, in Centralblatt, 1875, No. 14.

has recorded something similar) has observed that with newly born dogs the excitation of regions corresponding to the psycho-motor points produces no muscular movement in the corresponding limbs, whereas, some time after birth, towards the ninth or eleventh days, these points become excitable.

These observations, though yet few, should nevertheless be taken into account, and they would seem to indicate that the psycho-motor centres are not pre-established, if one can so speak, so much anatomically as they are physiologically. They are developed by age, doubtless through functional exercise.

In support of this view I offer a remark with which I will terminate the special subject that has detained us. The regions of the large cells belong to the five-layer type, and these regions have no definite anatomical characteristic except the presence of giant-cells. Now these giant-cells, morphologically, do not differ essentially from the large pyramidal cells, which also, according to the researches of Koschewnikoff, possess, like them, the nerve-prolongations in addition to the protoplasmic prolongations, attributed to motor cells.

It seems natural to inquire if these cells, and even those of the smaller species, which are their miniature representatives, would not be capable, under certain conditions—under the influence, for example, of abnormal functional excitement—of acquiring development, and in that way giving birth to supplementary motor centres destined to replace primitive centres that by some lesion may have been destroyed. Thus, for example, might be explained how voluntary movements can be restored in a part, notwithstanding the destruction of a motor centre—a phenomenon, an example of which is furnished in the frequent recovery from aphasia, in despite of the persistence of the lesion of the third frontal convolution.

D. To complete the examination of the cerebral cortex, I have but to add some little information upon its peculiarities in the posterior region of the brain.

These peculiarities belong to the entire occipital lobe, the sphenoidal lobe, and the posterior and median parts of the hemisphere to the posterior border of the quadrilateral lobule.

The general character of the gray substance in those regions is that the pyramidal nerve-cells, as a rule, are very scarce and small, while the granular, on the contrary, are notably predominant. It is not that there are no large nerve-cells, but they are comparatively rare—*solitary*, to employ the expression of Meynert. Betz adds that they have no nerve-prolongations, and that even the protoplasmic prolongations are scarcely developed.

The portion of the brain where this peculiarity is to be observed corresponds, according to many authors, to the *sensorium commune*. If this interpretation be correct, it would follow that the cells of which we are about to speak are cells of sensation. This hypothesis rests upon still other anatomical considerations, and upon pathological evidence of which I will hereafter give more detail.

FOURTH LECTURE.

PARALLEL BETWEEN SPINAL AND CEREBRAL LESIONS.

Summary :—The Indispensable Conditions for the Study of Cerebral
Localization in Diseases in Man.—Necessity of Good Clinical Observations and Regular Autopsy.—Natural History of Encephalic Lesions.
—Parallel between the Grand Compartments of the Cerebro-spinal
Axis.—Systemization of Lesions in the Spinal Cord.—Spinal Localizations.—The Brain is placed under a Pathological Regime Differing
from other Parts of the Nerve-Axis; Rarity of Localizations.—Difference of Lesions.—Frequency of Vascular Lesions in Maladies of the
Brain.—Necessity of the Study of Vascular Distribution.—Outline of
the Cerebral Arteries.

GENTLEMEN :

From the preceding lectures you comprehend that, unprepared by a precise knowledge of normal anatomy, it would be
useless to undertake this subject.

The subordination of pathological to normal anatomy is
most especially obvious in all questions related to cerebral
pathology. This will directly be rendered still more evident.

I. To-day we will commence by recounting the indispensable conditions for solving the problems connected with *localization in cerebral diseases*, as exhibited in man.

The following are the fundamental ones : 1st. A good clinical observation made with the most complete possible knowledge of existing facts in experimental physiology. 2d. A
regular, anatomically precise autopsy.

Our preceding topographical studies make an important
step, for they will better enable us to determine the locations,
extent, and configuration of lesions revealed by autopsy.

For the special object which we have in view, however,
even the most minute and exact anatomical observations can-

3

not always be utilized. Here as elsewhere, it is necessary
that observation should teach us how to select from things
seen, and in this process more than one difficulty must be
overcome.

To make you familiar with the situation it is best first to
survey the *natural history of encephalic lesions*.

1st. What are the alterations capable of affecting the encephalon, or especially the brain? We are now, of course,
dealing only with the most usual forms of cerebral disease—
with partial or circumscribed lesions as they are called; such
only can be profitably considered in this connection.

2d. In the second place, what are the general anatomical
conditions which preside either at the development, or during the process of reparation of such lesions? For there is
no chance work, even in the encephalon.

To accomplish our end I propose once more to employ the
comparative method, that lever so powerful in natural sci-
ences. I will make, pathologico-anatomically, a comparison
between the grand cerebro-spinal compartments (or if you
choose Piorry's nomenclature, *nerve-axis*); that is: 1st, the
spinal cord; 2d, the *rachidian bulb;* 3d, the *brain proper.*

A. It may be said that the pathological physiology of the
spinal cord is distinguished by the extensive existence in it
of those lesions called *systemic.* By this expression, borrowed from Vulpian, are meant those lesions which are sys-
temically (the term is perfectly appropriate) circumscribed,
and which do not overstep the limits of certain clearly determined regions in that complex organ. I beg to refer you to
figure No. 21, which will recall our past lectures.

You remember that there are lesions limited to the anterior
cornua of the gray substance (Fig. 7). They are, in acute
form, infantile paralysis; in chronic form, the various kinds
of progressive locomotor ataxia. There are other lesions
limited to the lateral fasciculi and which are distinguished by
symptoms of numbness (paresic) with a tendency to contractions. You know that the fibres of Goll may alone be subject to lesions; and that the regions of the little external bands
(Fig. 7) (*posterior columns*) in the area of the lateral fasciculi

is the only anatomical *substratum* necessary for symptoms of spinal tabes.

It is thus that pathological anatomy, guided in its first steps by experiment with animals, and aided also by clinical experience, has become able to separate, in man, the complex organ called the spinal cord, into a certain number of compartments, departments, and secondary organs.

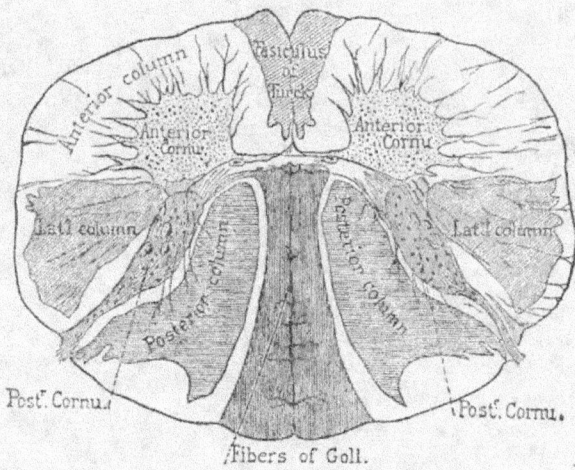

FIG. 7.—Transverse section of spinal cord.

To each systemic lesion of these various regions belong groups of symptoms or syndromes which clinically serve to individualize them, and which have also given place, in pathological descriptions of the spinal cord, to a certain number of *elementary affections*. Analysis, founded upon a knowledge of the elementary affections, is a great help in unveiling mixed or complex forms.

The study of these systemic lesions has doubtless contributed greatly to rescue *spinal localization* from its past chaos.

B. Systemic lesions are found extended to the *rachidian bulb*, the *protuberance*, and the *crura cerebri*. I will cite for examples the *secondary degenerations* of the cord consecutive to lesions of the brain, *primitive* and *symmetrical sclerosis* of the *lateral column*, *bulbous paralysis* from exclusive lesion of the ganglia at the origin of the nerves, etc. But above that point this mode of *pathological alteration* does not appear to exist, and it may be said that to the present *systemic lesions* in the brain are unknown.

No one really knows of *systemic lesions* limited to the thalami optici, to the different ganglia of the corpora striata, or to the various portions of the cortex. It does not follow, however, that strict research cannot determine *anatomical localizations* in the encephalon, but they are at present relatively rare, and seemingly accidental.

What is the real reason of this singular fact ? It is that the *encephalon* is placed under a *pathological régime, so to speak, differing from that controlling other portions of the nerve-axis.* In fact, speaking in a general way, in the encephalon, and especially in the brain, the vascular system (arteries, veins, and capillaries) commands the situation.

I will call attention to the importance of vascular ruptures and ensuing hemorrhage in the intra-encephalic centres; the predominant rôle of vascular obliterations by thromboses and emboli, the effect of which is extravasation followed by partial softening of the brain.

I will enumerate the most common anatomical causes of organic disease in the encephalon.

C. If we now return to the spinal cord and bulb, we will observe a remarkable contrast to the encephalon. Hemorrhage by vascular rupture, whether resulting from the alteration well known under the name of *miliary aneurism*, from softening consecutive to arterial narrowing, or from thrombosis or embolism, is something which in the spinal cord is almost unknown.

The bulb constitutes, as it were, the transition between the spinal cord and the encephalon, for in the bulb is seen, on the one hand, *systemic lesions* which recall those seen in the cord, and on the other hand, a certain number of hemorrhages and softenings are found resulting from vascular lesions.

These last, however, are still more frequent in the protuberance, the pathology of which also approaches more nearly that of the encephalon. Hemorrhage from rupture of miliary aneurism, and softening by vascular obliteration, here become frequent.

D. These considerations explain why the most common *anatomical localization* in the encephalon is to be arrived at chiefly through a knowledge of the vascular distribution ; for the broken vessel being known, one can, as Lépine has truly said, decide the outline and extent of the territory involved.

This directs us once more to the field of normal anatomy, for the purpose of obtaining some general ideas relative to the vascularization of the encephalon. This is a subject worthy of your entire attention, the more so that the questions relating thereto have been thoroughly investigated, and to this your countrymen have contributed their share.

II. For the present it will suffice to examine the arterial system, although lesions of the venous system have also a marked influence upon the development of encephalic alterations. The immediate object is to show by some examples how important a profound knowledge of the normal conditions of cerebral circulation is to the understanding of the majority of anatomical lesions of the brain.

You remember the manner in which the trunks of the two internal carotids and the two vertebral arteries join at the base of the encephalon to carry on the circulation.[1]

The internal carotids, as they leave the cavernous sinus, run

---

[1] It is known that hemorrhage and softening of the brain are much more frequent on the left than on the right side. Duret, in his *mémoire*, thinks to have discovered the anatomical solution of this fact in the manner in which the primitive carotid and the vertebral arteries of the left side originate. The right carotid arises from the innominate, and the innominate, at a considerable angle, from the axis of the aorta, whereas the left carotid ascends nearly perpendicularly, and its axis is more nearly continuous with the ascending aorta. It follows that a clot expelled by a cardiac contraction would, by a direct line, be more apt to enter the left carotid. The right vertebral artery rises from the horizontal portion of the subclavian after it has made its curve ; the left vertebral artery, on the contrary, takes its rise from the summit of the curve of the subclavian.

perpendicularly to the base of the brain, and immediately divide into two branches, the one anterior (the *anterior cerebral*), the other, running laterally, bears the name of *Sylvian, or middle cerebral artery* (Fig. 8). Near their origin the two anterior cerebral arteries are transversely united, and thus, in a more or less complete manner, the circulation of the two internal carotids are unified. That vascular arrangement con-

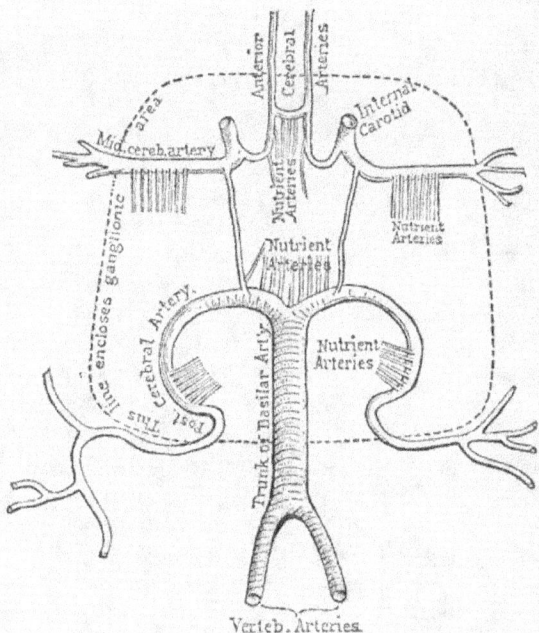

{ FIG. 8.—Scheme of arterial circulation at the base of the encephalon.

stitutes a special system, to which may be given the name of anterior system, or *carotid system*.

The *vertebral* arteries, directed obliquely from behind forward, converge towards the median line and unite in a single trunk, the *basilar trunk*. Towards the anterior border of the protuberance, this basilar trunk separates into two branches, called the *posterior cerebral arteries*, and these constitute a second arterial system, the posterior, or *vertebral system*.

The *carotid system* and the *vertebral system*, united by two vessels called the posterior communicants, and which are quite variable in volume and arrangement,[1] form a vascular circle at the base of the brain, known to all anatomists under the name of the hexagonal, or better, the *polygon of Willis*.

At the anterior angles of the polygon of Willis are the two anterior cerebral arteries; from the antero-lateral angles, running outwards, arise the two Sylvian (middle cerebral) arteries, and finally, the posterior angle is formed by the posterior cerebral arteries. This is the circle of Willis, and the first two centimètres of those various arterial trunks give rise to the nutrient arteries of the central ganglia, the corpora striata and thalami optici.

There are six principal groups of these nutrient arteries.

The first—*antero-median group*—has its origin in the anterior communicant and in the commencement of the anterior cerebral arteries. The arterioles of which it is composed nourish the anterior part of the head of the caudated ganglion.

The second—*postero-median group*—arises from the posterior half of the posterior communicants, and from the origin of the posterior cerebral arteries. They nourish the internal face of the thalami optici and the walls of the third ventricle.

The third and fourth—*right and left antero-lateral groups*—composed of a larger number of arterioles, rise from the Sylvian arteries and supply the corpora striata and the *anterior* part of the thalami optici.

The fifth and sixth—*postero-lateral groups*—are derived from the posterior cerebral arteries after they have passed around the crura cerebri; they nourish a great part of the thalami optici.

A line surrounding the circle of Willis, two centimètres out-

---

[1] Duret has directed attention to the frequent variations and anomalies of the circle of Willis and the communicants. These last are often filiform and entirely insufficient to re-establish circulation in case of obliterations. Certain forms of anomalies explain also cases of softening of an *entire* hemisphere, by a clot obliterating the internal carotid near its bifurcation.

side of it, would include the origin of the *ganglionic* arteries, and it might also be termed the *ganglionic circle* (Fig. 8).

The cortical regions (the convolutions of the cerebral hemispheres) are irrigated by the large arteries which form the angles and sides of the circle of Willis.

The *anterior cerebral artery* winds around the corpus callosum, and spreads upon a portion of the inferior face of the anterior or frontal lobe (*gyrus rectus and gyri supra-orbitales*) and over a larger portion of the internal face of the hemisphere (*first and second frontal convolutions, præcentral and quadrilateral or præcuneus lobules.*)

The *posterior cerebral artery*, springing from the basilar, winds around the corresponding cerebral peduncle, and divides into three branches, which go to the inferior face of the brain and to the occipital lobe (*gyrus uncinatus ; gyrus hippocampi ; second, third and fourth temporal convolutions ; the cuneus ; lobulus lingualis*).

The Sylvian (middle cerebral) artery is distributed to that part of the frontal lobe which is not vascularized by the anterior cerebral artery, and over the entire parietal lobe. Later it will be necessary to follow in detail the distribution of each of the four branches of this important artery, and to describe exactly their vascular territories.

Such, then, is the general distribution of the arteries sent to the internal, external, and inferior faces of the brain. To understand the interior vascular arrangement it is necessary to have recourse to various sections. Upon a single section made within the domain of the Sylvian artery, the circulation in the gray ganglia will seem to be confounded with that of the surrounding gray matter and the subjacent white ganglia ; that is but an illusion, however, which will be dispelled in the next lecture.

FIFTH AND SIXTH LECTURES.

ARTERIAL CIRCULATION IN THE BRAIN.

Summary:—Labors of Duret and Heubner.—Principal Arteries of the Brain.—The System of Cortical Arteries.—Nutrient Vessels.—System of the Central Arteries, or of the Central Ganglia.—Sylvian Artery; Its Branches; Arteries of the Central Gray Ganglia; Cortical Branches; Ramifications and Arborizations; Nutrient Arteries of the Encephalic Pulp; they are Long (Medullary Arteries) and Short (Cortical Arteries).—Effects of Obliterations of the Various Arteries. —Superficial Softenings, Yellow Spots.—Communication between the Vascular Territories; Opinion of Heubner; Opinion of Duret.—Terminal Arteries (Cohnheim).—Relative Autonomy of the Vascular Territories of the Brain.—Localizations of Cortical Lesions.—Branches of the Sylvian Artery; Frontal, External, and Inferior.—Artery of the Ascending Frontal Convolution.—Artery of the Ascending Parietal Convolution.—Artery of the Gyrus Angularis.—Anterior and Posterior Cerebral Arteries; their Branches.

GENTLEMEN:

To-day I propose to examine more thoroughly the subject which was barely introduced in our last lecture. If I have clearly shown that in cerebral pathology it is the arterial system which commands the situation, I must, as a matter of course, through the same effort, have proved the necessity of preliminary studies concerning the physiological connection between the circulation and the various departments that compose the brain proper.

How, indeed, can one comprehend the *rationale* of hemorrhagic centres, or centres of softening, which constitute the chief pathological anatomy of the brain, if he is not entirely familiar with the special distribution of the arterial vessels, an alteration in which is the commencement or the first condition of these various lesions.

Unapplied facts in normal anatomy will not here suffice. But the application of them at once suggests itself. I have

already shown this, and I shall now exhibit it still more
clearly.

I pause at this point in the anatomy of cerebral circulation, because that, even in the works most justly esteemed,
you will find on this subject only the most vague and entirely insufficient information, quite inadequate to our needs.

All the precise knowledge which we have is of recent date,
and is the result of studies exacted through the needs of
pathological anatomy and physiology.

I shall borrow particularly from the important work of our
countryman, Duret—a work which has been executed in the
laboratory of Salpêtrière. Duret has encountered a rival in
his field. That rival is a German doctor, Heubner, professor
at the Leipzig University. These two authors, unacquainted
with each other, have pursued their researches simultaneously,
and in the most essential points they have arrived at identical results. That assuredly is a guarantee of the exactness
of the descriptions which they have given us.

In a recent work treating of syphilitic alterations in the
cerebral arteries,[1] Heubner professes to have been the initia-
tor. That is a claim which cannot be sustained. The first
researches of Duret relative to the circulation in the bulb and
the protuberance were communicated to the *Société de Bio-
logie* in the session of Dec. 7, 1872.

By a remarkable coincidence, the same day, the 7th of
December, the *résumé* of the researches of Heubner upon
cerebral circulation was published at Berlin in the *Centralblatt.* One month after, in January, 1873, Duret published
a note in the *Progrès médical*[2] concerning that part of his
researches which treated also of the cerebral circulation. The
investigations of Duret are not, then, two years later than
those of Heubner, as the latter insinuates ; they are exactly
contemporaneous. Of this fact Heubner might easily have
convinced himself, as he has become acquainted with the last
mémoire of Duret, published in the *Archives de physiolo-*

---

[1] Die luetische Erkrankung der Hirnarterien, p. 188, Leipzig, 1874.
[2] 18th and 25th of January, 1st of February, 8th and 15th of November, 1873.

gie (1874), where the history of the question is given in detail.[1]

I have thought it well to insist upon this chronology, in face of the annexation mania, in order to establish the large part which belongs to our countryman.

I. I come to the special object of our studies. You know the manner in which the three trunks, rising from the circle of Willis, divide among themselves the arterial circulation in each cerebral hemisphere. They are : 1st, the anterior cerebral ; 2d, the middle cerebral or Sylvian artery, each rising from the internal carotid ; 3d, the posterior cerebral, branches from the basilar, a single trunk formed by the confluence of the two vertebral arteries.

A. Each one of these arteries, in each hemisphere, commands a special province ; I have already briefly acquainted you with the general topography and limits of these main vascular territories, and they should be examined not only at the surface of the hemispheres, but also, by aid of sections, in their interiors.

Our attention should first be given to the surface of the brain, including the external, superior, internal, and inferior faces, and secondly to frontal sections, which will demonstrate the preponderating importance of the Sylvian territory.

We will soon see that these territories or provinces can be divided into a certain number of secondary departments, corresponding to the distribution of so many secondary arteries emanating from the principal trunks.

B. Without stopping longer at this first general view, we will enter at once into details. Each one of the three principal arteries gives rise to two very different systems of secondary vessels. The first of these may be denominated the *system of cortical arteries.* The vessels of which it is com-

---

[1] The researches of Duret possess a considerable pathological interest, for they have been made especially to explain the appearance of lesions found in autopsies. With the aid of more than two hundred cases furnished him by Charcot, he has been able to establish an anatomical classification of cerebral hemorrhages and softenings.

posed are spread through the pia mater, and there divide, after a peculiar method, before furnishing the little vessels which penetrate the cerebral pulp, and which are really the *nutrient vessels* of the gray matter and the subjacent medullary substance.

The second system is the *central system*, or the *system of the cerebral ganglia (gray central masses)*. The vessels of which it is composed rise from each of the three principal arteries close to their origin, and, in the form of arterioles, plunge immediately into the substance of the ganglionic masses.

The two systems, although they have a common origin, are entirely independent of each other, and at the border of their domains they have no point of intercommunication.

C. We must study the two systems in each of the main vascular territories. In doing this we will observe both common and special traits. We will first examine the Sylvian artery, the most important and the most complicated of the three cerebral arteries ; after that the description of the two others will be simple.

II. The Sylvian artery enters the fissure of Sylvius, the lips of which must be separated in order to bring the vessel well in view. But before this it furnishes from its superior border, in a region called the *anterior perforated space (locus perforatus anticus)*, a series of arteries which, running parallel to each other, enter each of the channels of the perforated space, which space is composed of the white substance (*substantia perforata*). These are the *arteries of the central gray ganglia*, or more definitely, *the arteries of the corpora striata*. Let us here examine the cortical system, leaving for the moment the gray ganglia.

At the bottom of the fissure of Sylvius is seen the island of Reil, on a level with which the Sylvian artery divides into four branches, each of which deserves a special name. These branches follow the furrows that separate the convolutions of the island and to which they furnish vessels. They then bend inwards and outwards, and rise again to the surface of the hemisphere, where they are distributed, as we have just said, over a certain number of fundamental convolutions, where they form a number of little secondary territories corresponding to each one of the convolutions.   (Fig. 9.)

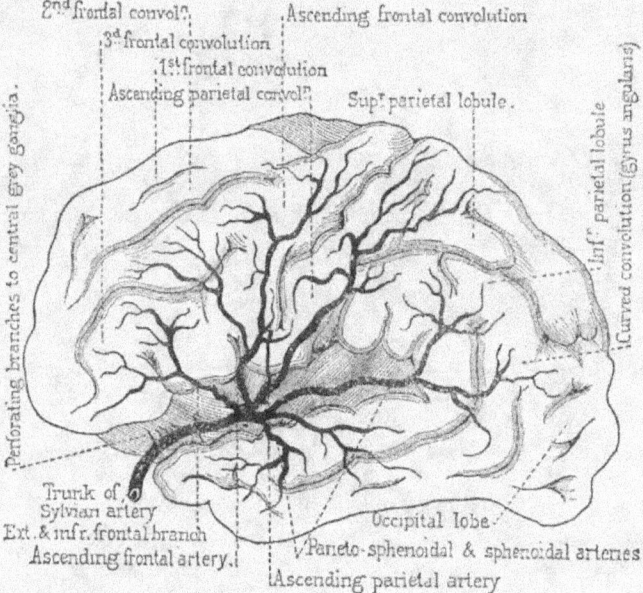

FIG. 9.—Distribution of Sylvian artery.   (*Partially schematic.*)

We will not dwell, however, upon this description, but proceed to examine more thoroughly the manner in which the cortical arteries are divided and distributed to the substance of the pia mater before they penetrate the cerebral pulp.

I should mention that the branches arising from the Sylvian artery immediately subdivide into branches of the third order, to the number of two or three for each secondary trunk.   These *tertiary* branchlets constitute a kind of vascular skeleton, upon which is grafted a system of *arborizations;* that is a special and very original system of small vessels, which arise not only from the extremities of the branches, but also from the trunks themselves.

Contrary to the assertions of most authors, Duret affirms that these arborizations do not anastomose with each other, although the branchlets sometimes communicate with those of the neighboring territories.   (Fig. 10.)

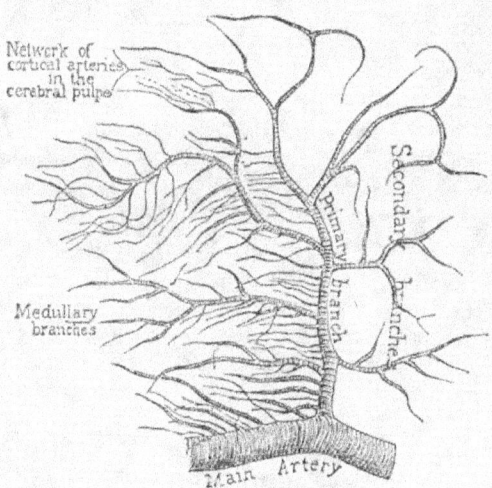

Fig. 10.—Arterial division in the encephalon.   (*Duret.*)

The *ramifications* and *arborizations* are on a plane with the pia mater. On the internal face of that membrane they give off the *nutrient arteries*, which enter the encephalic pulp perpendicularly.   The nutrient vessels here are all, according to the definition of Ch. Robin, capillaries.   This character distinguishes them from the vessels of the central ganglia, which bury themselves in the white substance of the base of the brain (anterior perforated space), inasmuch as these last retain the structure and dimensions of arteries.

By aid of sections which can be examined microscopically, we will now investigate more closely the peculiarities of these *nutrient arteries*.

Upon section of an entire convolution, made perpendicularly to the surface, there appears, first at the periphery, the gray substance which is like a festoon, having a thickness of two or three millimètres; next to this is the medullary substance composed of diverging and commissural fibres, binding one convolution to another. In such sections what is found to be the arrangement of the arteries? There can easily be distinguished two kinds of nutrient arteries which have long since been recognized by many authors, and particularly by Todd and Bowman. Of these arteries one kind are *long* and the other *short*.

1st. The *long arteries*, otherwise called the *medullary arteries*, arise from the *ramifications*, or indeed are the terminals of the *arborizations*. A dozen or fifteen may be seen upon a section of a convolution; three or four at the free surface; the others distributed upon the two slopes or in the separating furrow. The arteries at the summit are vertical—one of them generally occupies the middle part of the convolution; the arteries on the slope are oblique; those which occupy the bottom of the furrow are again vertical. These arteries penetrate the centrum ovale to the depth of three or four centimètres; they proceed without intercommunicating, except by means of fine capillaries, and in that way constitute so many little independent systems. At their terminations they approach the extremities of the central system of arteries, *but there is no communication whatever between the two systems.*

Thus there exists upon the confines of the two domains a sort of neutral ground where nutrition is less active. This neutral ground is more especially the location of *lacunal senile softenings*.

2d. The *short nutrient or cortical arteries* have the same origin as the long ones, but they are finer and shorter, and end, so to speak, on the road. Some run to the inner border of the gray layer, to the edge of the medullary centre; others are of less extent, and terminate in the gray substance. These short arteries give rise to capillary vessels which, conjoined with those emanating from the long arteries, form a mesh or web.

In the convolutions this network possesses the following characters (Fig. 11): 1st. The first layer has the thickness of a half millimètre; it is but slightly vascularized; 2d. The second layer corresponds to two zones of nerve-cells; there the vascular network is very compact, and with very fine polygonal interspaces; 3d. At the edge of that layer the interspaces become larger; 4th. Finally, in the medullary substance the interspaces become still larger and vertically elongated.

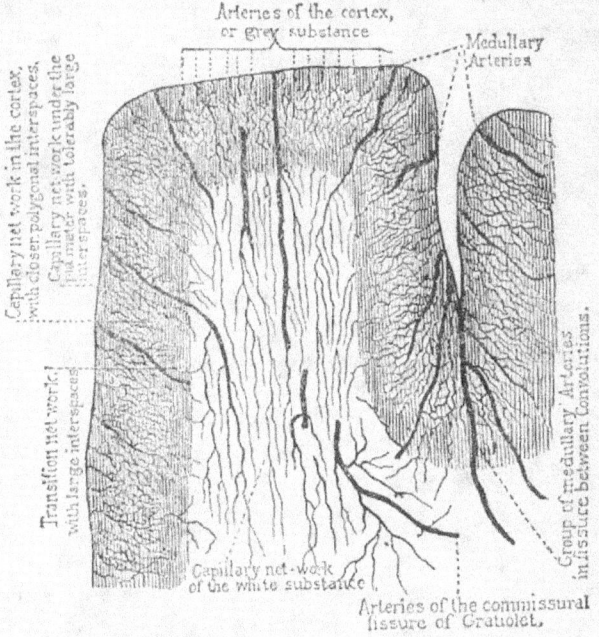

FIG. 11.—Arterial distribution in the cerebral cortex.

From the preceding facts it follows that, as concerns the arterial distribution, the gray and subjacent white cortex are a unit, since the vessels which they receive are derived in common from the arteries which traverse the pia mater. Should these last be obliterated at a given point, the gray and white substance would suffer simultaneously in the corresponding parts, and would be subject to that kind of mortification called *ischæmic cerebral softening*. The reciprocal relations of the parts permit a scheme of superficial softenings.

Recall the general distribution of the nutrient vessels. They are directed parallel to each other like so many lines towards the central parts. The white and the gray regions of the cortex can then, as vascular departments, be divided into a number of wedges, the bases of which are directed towards the encephalon, and the apices towards the central parts. This is, indeed, the form assumed by the greater number of those softenings called *superficial*. That at once calls to mind the appearance of infarctus of the spleen and kidney. If the softening is an old one—that is, of several weeks' standing—the gray substance appears depressed in consequence of the destruction of its elements and the concomitant turning up of the subjacent white substance.

The superficial portions of the softening produce a *yellow spot*. The yellow color belongs exclusively to the gray substance, the subjacent softened white substance being only blanched, or sometimes lightly tinted with yellow.

A. In this case we have supposed the obliteration of a branch of the second or third order. The obliteration of the trunk of the Sylvian artery itself might produce necrosis of all the gray cortex and of the subjacent white cortex also.

The central parts would be entirely spared if the obliteration occurred above the origin of the arteries of the *corpora striata*.

B. It need not be supposed that all obliterations of this kind would necessarily and surely produce such disastrous effects. There are rare cases where, in fact, such obliteration of a branch of the Sylvian artery, or even the artery itself (I here take the Sylvian artery as example, it would be the same for the *anterior* or *posterior cerebral* arteries)—there are cases, I say, in which the obliteration in question has no appreciable, or, at least, but passing results.

If this be so, it follows that the three main vascular territories into which the brain is divided, and the departments into which they in turn are separated, are not strictly isolated, individual territories. They may communicate, and indeed do communicate in the ordinary manner. But are these communications easy and constant, or, on the contrary, are

4

they accidental, indirect, and often impracticable ? In the solution of this question authors are at variance.

Heubner holds that the communications in question are very easy, that they are made by the mediation of vessels not less than a millimètre in diameter. He rests that assertion upon the results of injections, where he has invariably observed that the material injected into any one of the departments by the principal trunk, or by the branches, always rapidly penetrates the other territories.

He also cites pathological cases which indicate that obliteration of one of the vessels of the cortical system or of its branches has, during life, given no evident symptom ; cases in which death having followed, the cerebral pulp in the parts corresponding to the obliteration has at autopsy presented no trace of softening.

In the first place, as to the pathological facts of Heubner, we must recognize that they are real ; of this there is no doubt. At the same time, to judge from the very numerous observations which I have collected, they are certainly rare.

On the other hand, it is certain that in anatomy things are far from being always as seen by Heubner. The observations of Duret in that field have been numerous, and are nearly always in accord.

Here is briefly what we learn from them :

Let ligatures be placed upon each of the three principal arteries at the base of the encephalon on both sides, immediately above their origin in the circle of Willis. Then inject the Sylvian artery. This will first fill the Sylvian territory, and in the majority of cases it will pass beyond its limits. The injected material invades the neighboring parts slowly, little by little. This invasion is made from the periphery inwards towards the centre of the invaded territory. It is effected through the mediation of vessels of small calibre belonging to the system of *ramifications* having diameters of but a quarter or a fifth of a millimètre, contrary to the opinion of Heubner, who holds that these anterial vessels have a diameter of one millimètre.

The number of anastomoses from territory to territory

are also quite variable. There are cases where one of the three grand territories can be injected isolatedly, the anastomoses not being sufficient to permit the injection to enter the adjacent territories. The communication which may occur at the periphery of a vascular territory explains why the obliteration of a main trunk often results in the softening of only the central parts of the territory, the peripheral portion remaining untouched.

Such are the conclusions of Duret, and to my mind they are more in conformity with pathological facts than those of Heubner. I should add that Cohnheim, who has also experimented in partial injections of the encephalic arteries, agrees with Duret. He says if the arteries of the encephalon are not *final* or *terminal* arteries (we will explain what Cohnheim means by that term), they very nearly approach that type.

Under the name of *terminal* or *final* arteries (Endarterien) Cohnheim[1] ingeniously catalogues those arteries or arterioles which, between their origin and the capillaries, neither furnish nor receive any anastomosing branch. An example of terminal arteries convenient for study is afforded by the tongue of the frog, upon which it is easy, through the microscope, to observe (*de visu*) all the effects of an obliteration. You see upon these schematic designs the various consequences of the obliteration of a terminal artery. The results are, as it were, certain. If, on the other hand, we deal with an anastomosing artery, generally the circulation is easily reestablished below the point of lesion, by means of anastomoses. But these anastomoses may in their turn be obliterated, and it so may follow that an artery which in its normal state is not at all a *terminal* artery, may become so by accident.

The encephalic circulation furnishes a great many examples of terminal arteries. Thus, without including the ramifications which exist in the pia mater, we can instance the nutrient arteries. We see, too, that the arteries of the central ganglia are entirely and rigorously constructed on that model. The same type is found in all other circulatory systems where

---

[1] Untersuchungen ueber die embolischen Processe. Berlin, 1872.

pathological or experimental lesions by vascular obliterations usually result in what is termed *infarctus*. Such are the spleen, the kidney, the lung, and the retina. None of the viscera—and this observation belongs to Cohnheim—where infarctus is not the rule, have the *terminal* mode of arterial distribution.

But we will return to the relative individualities of the vascular territories of the brain. Those individualities do not belong exclusively to the large territories ; they are found also in the secondary departments, which correspond to the ramifications of arteries of the second and third order. Between these regions of the secondary order, the same as with the larger ones, communications are possible, but generally are very difficult. It follows that obliteration of one of these secondary branches might have, and often does have, the effect of inducing limited mortification in the cortex. This is an important point in the study of cerebral localization. It might be that a lesion thus limited would exactly correspond to one of the convolutions, or to a group of convolutions, endowed with specific properties, manifesting themselves during life through special phenomena.

You can readily comprehend that strict localization of lesions of the cortex, produced by obliterations of arterial branches of the second or third order, would be an especially interesting study, when occurring in the Sylvian region. It is in that large field that experimentation tends to place the famous motor centres ; it is there also that clinical experience, aided by pathological anatomy, has located the faculty of articulate language.

So it is important that we should be well acquainted with the principal branches rising from the Sylvian artery, and closely examine their distribution in the fundamental convolutions of that region.

The Sylvian artery divides into, or at least gives rise to, four principal branches. The distribution of these branches has been carefully studied by Duret and by Heubner. (See Figs. 9 and 12.)

The first Duret calls *frontal-external and inferior*. That

is really the artery of the third frontal convolution (convolution of Broca). I have myself several times seen an obliteration of this arterial trunk produce a softening confined to the

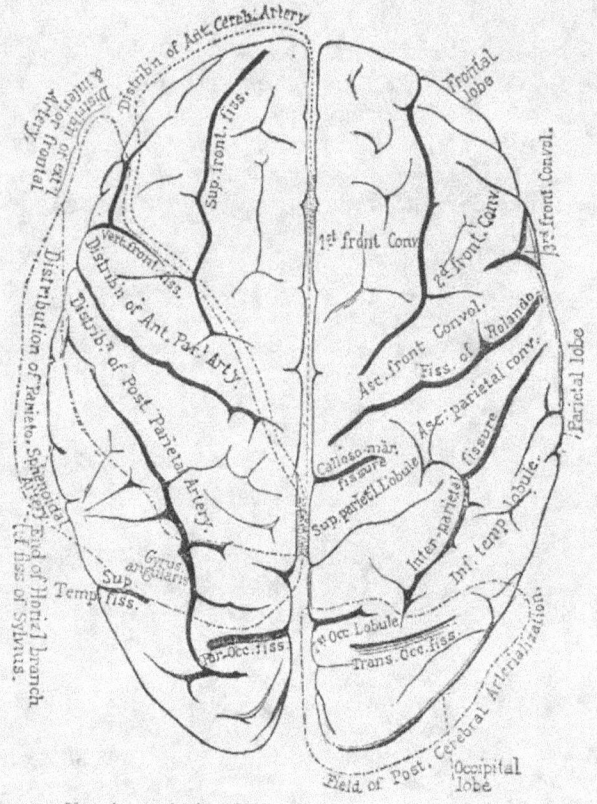

FIG. 12.—Vascular territories of the superior cerebral surface. (*Duret.*) The dotted lines indicate the territories of the anterior, middle and posterior arteries.

territory of the third convolution (in its posterior part). I here add a conclusively corroborative fact. The case was a woman named *Farn....* observed at Salpêtrière. She was attacked with aphasia. There had existed no trace of paralysis either of motion or sensation. Aphasia was in this case the only symptom, and atrophy of the third convolution was also the only corresponding lesion revealed by autopsy. (Figs. 13 and 14.) This is incontestably a fine example of cerebral localization.[1]

The *second branch* of the Sylvian is the *anterior parietal artery* of Duret. I prefer to term it the *artery of the ascending frontal convolution* (Fig. 9 and Fig. 12).

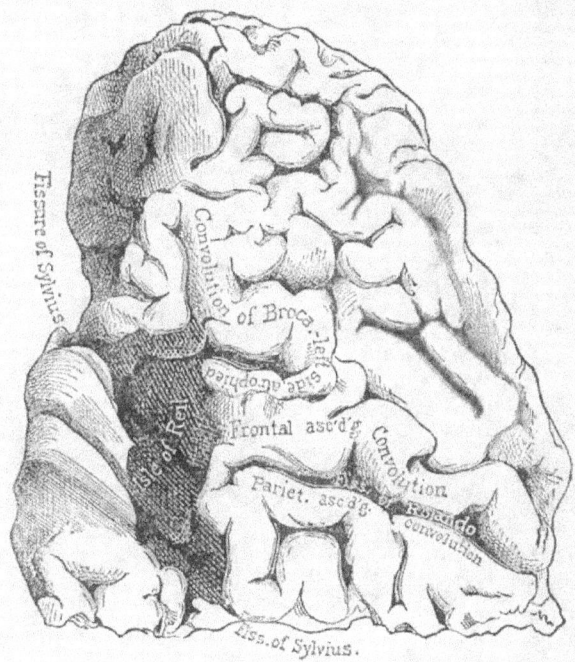

FIG. 13.—Human brain, anterior lobe, left side. (*Life size.*)

The third is the *posterior parietal artery*, which I think would be better named *artery* of the *ascending parietal convolution* (Fig. 9 and Fig. 12).

The fourth branch goes to the gyrus angularis and the first sphenoidal convolution (Fig. 9 and Fig. 12).

---

[1] We published the complete observations of that case in Nos. 20 and 21 of the *Progrès Médical*, 1874.

The two convolutions to which the second and third branches of the Sylvian artery are distributed furnish, according to the experiments of Ferrier upon the monkey, the motor centres of the limbs. You see that from the arterial distribution these two convolutions may suffer lesions independently of each other.

I do not know if the complete destruction of these two

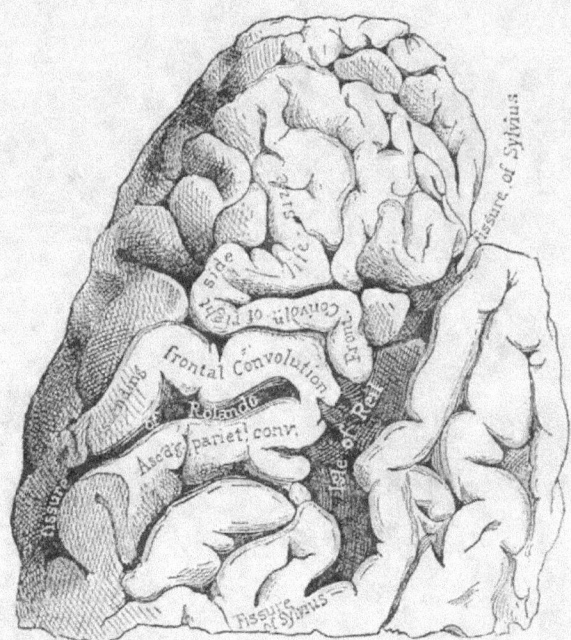

FIG. 14.—Human brain, anterior lobe, right side.   (*Life size.*)

central convolutions has ever been seen, but here is a case where entire destruction occurred of the ascending parietal convolution, which in the monkey is, according to Ferrier, the motor centre of the upper limbs, and partially so of the lower ones.

In this case the convolution in question was replaced by a depressed yellow spot. The frontal ascending convolution was not greatly altered, though it was manifestly atrophied. Now, though the thalami optici and the corpora striata were in that case uninjured—their integrity was very explicitly mentioned—there existed a complete and permanent hemiplegia in the upper and lower limbs of the opposite side (Fig. 15).

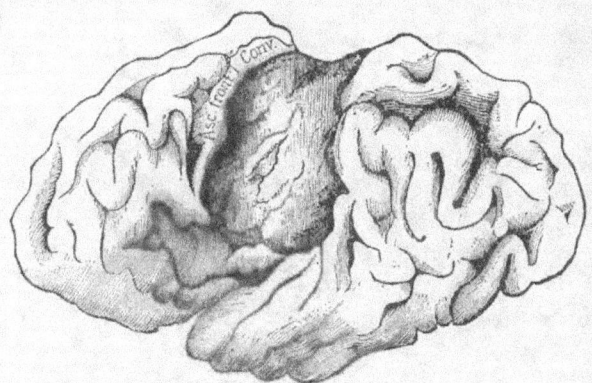

FIG. 15.—Human brain, left side ; destruction of the ascending parietal convolution and a great part of the frontal ascending convolution.

This is a result which contrasts singularly with those accompanying two other observations relative to extended lesions occupying other portions of the gray cortex of the brain. In one case of limited destruction of the quadrilateral lobule (yellow spot) there was no corresponding paralysis. In another case, there was also a yellow spot which included a large extent of the inferior face of the sphenoidal lobe, which you know is arterialized by the posterior cerebral artery. Here, also, in life there existed not a trace of hemiplegia.

I think these examples, which I could easily multiply, will suffice to convince you that some day not far in the future, it will be possible to surely establish in the human subject the doctrine of localization, at all events as concerns the superficial parts of the brain.

After the description which I have given respecting the Sylvian artery, I think I may be brief in that concerning the subdivision into secondary department of the main cortical vascular territories of the anterior and posterior cerebral arteries.

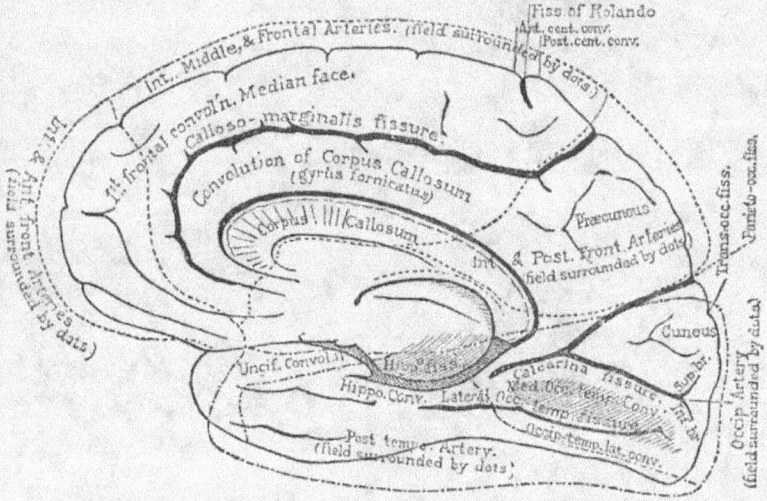

FIG. 16.—Vascular territories of the internal or median face of the human brain, indicated by the dotted lines.

III. The *anterior cerebral artery* is much less frequently the seat of serious alterations than the Sylvian. That fact is doubtless in part owing to the angle at which the Sylvian leaves the internal carotid artery (Figs. 12, 16, and 17).

This artery gives three principal branches : the *first* nourishes the two inferior frontal convolutions ; the *second*, much more important, is distributed (less commonly than the Sylvian, but much oftener than the anterior cerebral) to the gyrus fornicatus (Fig. 16), to the corpus callosum, to the first frontal convolution (internal and external faces), to the paracentral lobule and upon the convex face of the frontal lobe, to the first and second frontal convolutions (Fig. 17), and finally to the superior extremity of the ascending frontal convolution. The *third* branch of the anterior cerebral artery is sent to the quadrilateral lobule, which may be subject to lesions on its own account, as I have just now given you an example.

IV. The *posterior cerebral artery* (Figs. 12, 16, and 17) often suffers alterations by embolismus and thrombus.

Ischæmic softenings of the posterior lobes are much more common than with the anterior lobes.

The territory of this artery is divided into three secondary

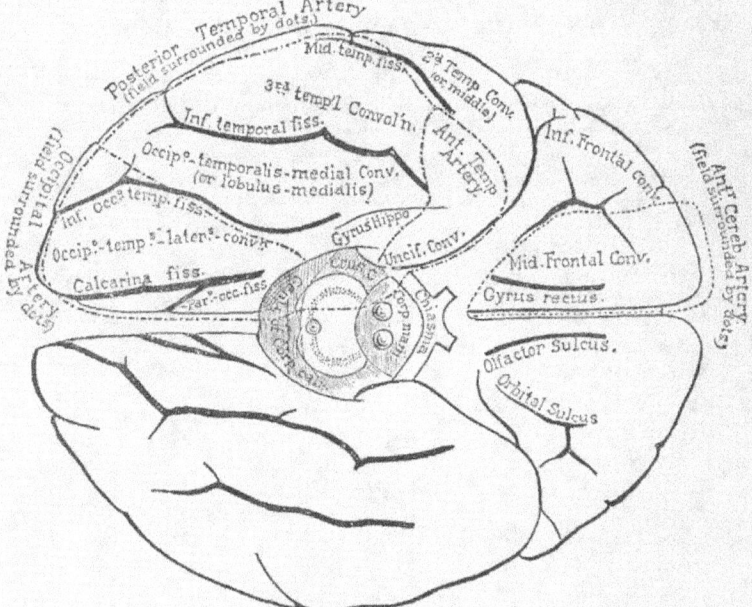

FIG. 17.—Vascular territories of the inferior face of the human brain, indicated by the dotted lines.

departments, corresponding to three arteries of the second order. The *first* of these goes to the gyrus angularis; the *second* to the inferior part of the sphenoidal lobe, embracing the inferior sphenoidal convolution and the fusiform lobule; the *third* goes to the lingual lobule, to the cuneus, and the occipital lobe proper.

SEVENTH LECTURE.

CIRCULATION IN THE CENTRAL MASSES (GRAY GANGLIA AND THE INTERNAL CAPSULE).

Summary:—Arterial Circulation in the Gray Central Ganglia; Intra-Encephalic Hemorrhage.—Anatomico-Pathological Differences between the Peripheral and Central Parts of the Brain.—Relative Infrequency of Cerebral Hemorrhage in the Peripheral Regions; its Frequency in the Central Parts.—Origin of the Arteries of the Central System.—Terminal Arteries; their Characters.—Independence of the Cortical and Central Arterial Systems.—Analogies between the Arteries of the Protuberance, the Bulb, and the Central Ganglia.—Their Mode of Origin Explains the Predominance in those Parts of Arterial Ruptures.—Branches Composing that System rise from the Anterior and Posterior Cerebral Arteries and the Sylvian Artery.—Arrangement of the Gray Ganglia; their Form and Relations.—Considerations upon the Internal Capsule; its Constituent Parts (Direct Peduncular Fasciculi, Indirect Peduncular Fasciculi, Diverging Fasciculi).

GENTLEMEN:

In the preceding lecture I concluded the anatomico-medical description of the cortical arterial system of the brain. I now purpose to call your attention to the arterial circulation in the *gray central ganglia*. Under this term are included the thalami optici, the corpora striata, and their so-called appendages. This is a study which should receive our closest care, for the phenomena which result from vascular lesions in these ganglia are clinically of no less importance than those which come from alterations in the arterial system of the superficial or cortical parts of the hemispheres. We will find in these central parts of the brain ischæmic alterations such as belong to its superficial layers; but, besides these, we will there find, and upon a larger scale, lesions which are rare upon the periphery. I refer to common *intra-ence-*

phalic hemorrhage, one of the most constant anatomical causes of those symptoms signified by the term *apoplexy*.

In this connection there exists a difference sufficiently interesting to be noticed between the peripheral and central parts of the brain. In the periphery, intra-encephalic hemorrhage is relatively rare, whereas in the centre it is common. This is a fact of which the statistics of Andral and Durand-Fardel are eloquent witnesses, and they are confirmed by recent statistics. Thus, of 119 cases collected by Andral and Durand-Fardel, the thalami optici and corpora striata have been found the original seat of hemorrhage in 102 cases; in only 17 cases has the hemorrhagic origin been either in the anterior or posterior lobe or at the periphery of the brain. On the other hand, ischæmic softenings of the brain predominate, as Durand-Fardel truly says, in the periphery. The facts which I have gathered at Salpêtrière in every point confirm these statements.

We will presently indicate some of the conditions necessary to explain this remarkable contrast; just now it is sufficient to convince you that our review of the *corticular arterial* system was a necessary introduction to the chapter upon ischæmic softenings of the brain; the studies which will occupy us to-day furnish the obligatory preface of the equally interesting history of intra-encephalic hemorrhage.

I. You remember how the arterioles of the central system are derived from the three great arterial trunks of the brain, near their origin in the circle of Willis. The arteries which form the central system are generally vessels of some size. For the corpora striata they are, according to Duret, arterioles measuring in diameter from a half to one and a half millimètres.

Their mode of origin calls to mind the shoots rising from the base of forest trees. I borrow the comparison from Heubner, which, beyond its picturesque character, is quite true; only it must not be carried too far, for the arteries of the central system, at their point of departure, take a direction perpendicular to the principal trunk.

This perpendicular direction brings to mind that which we have noticed respecting the nutrient arteries of the cortex. But it is well not to forget that there is a difference between the nutrient cortical vessels and the arteries of the gray central ganglia; the first, indeed, are but capillaries—at least as defined by Robin—and the second, on the contrary, are vessels of larger size.

Another character belonging to the arteries of the central ganglia is that (as the term is used by Cohnheim) they are *terminal arteries par excellence.* If the independency of the vascular territories of the cortex is, as we have seen, open to discussion, it is not the same respecting the central arteries. Authors fully agree that they are entirely independent of each other.

Thus Heubner says that by the aid of a Pravaz syringe (its point blunted) one can inject each of the small arteries that lead to the various parts of the corpora striata and thalami optici. With all possible precautions, however, one can never inject the entire body of the thalamus opticus or corpus striatum. Only small departments of each can be injected, and if the injection is made too forcibly, ruptures are produced; but notwithstanding that, the vascular territories keep to their assigned limits.

The multiplied experiences of Duret are to the same effect. It should be added that *under no circumstances can an injection be passed by way of the central arteries into the domain of the cortical arteries,* and the reverse is equally true—the central system cannot be injected through the cortical.

It is perhaps not without interest to notice the analogies in the manner in which the nutrient arteries originate in the basilar parts of the encephalon, in the protuberance, and even in the bulb.

In the *protuberance* the resemblance is striking; the median arteries leave the voluminous basilar artery at right angles and penetrate to the posterior part of the protuberance parallel to each other and without anastomosing, reproducing somewhat the type of terminal arteries.

In the *bulb* the same method exists, but somewhat differing through a special modification. The median arteries of the bulb do not rise immediately from the great trunks of the vertebral arteries ; they have their origin in the spinal arteries.

This mode of origin and distribution of the arteries of the protuberance and the central ganglia, possibly explains one of the reasons (a mechanical one) of the predominance in those parts of arterial rupture.

Remember that at the surface of the brain, where, as I have said, hemorrhages are comparatively rare, the arteries are not admitted to the pulp except after a long journey through the pia mater, and after being transformed into very slender vessels, in fact capillaries—recall, I say, these peculiarities, and you will much more easily comprehend the differences which I have pointed out to you concerning the central arteries.

1st. The distance from the heart to the large ganglia of the base is very short. The arteries supplying these ganglia come directly from the arteries forming the circle of Willis, that is, from arteries of the third order from the heart. This is evidently favorable to arterial ruptures. To be sure, this is obviated to a certain degree by the right angle at the origin of the vessels, and also by a considerable reduction of calibre.

2d. Compared with the cortical arteries, the central are voluminous ; I allude especially to the arteries of the corpora striata, which have a diameter of one-half to one and a half millimètres.

3d. I would add that the absence of anastomosis seems an unfortunate condition, for in case of increased pressure in a vessel, the clearing of the way is impossible on account of the absence of well-established collaterals.

The three great arterial trunks of the brain all take part in the vascularization of the central regions, but that participation is very unequal. The *anterior cerebral*, for example, sends only a few vessels to the head of the corpus striatum, and even these inconstantly. The *posterior cerebral artery* has a domain much more vast and important. It supplies the thalami optici, and to a great extent the superior portion of the crura cerebri and the tubercula quadrigemina. But here, as in the cortical system, the Sylvian arteries incontestably play the preponderating rôle. These arteries furnish all the branches which go to the caudated ganglion (with the exception of a little field of variable branches from the anterior cerebral) and to the various segments of the lenticular ganglion.

We will consequently take the branches of the Sylvian artery for the type of our description. After that, it will be easy to complete the description of the central nutrient system with the addition of a few words concerning some branches, derived, as may chance, from either the anterior or posterior cerebral arteries.

II. But before entering into the detailed description of these vessels it is very necessary to examine more closely than we have hitherto done the parts to which they are distributed. In the preceding description we have done little else than to name the parts, and in a summary manner to indicate their general configuration. That rapid notice is insufficient. We must enter into such examinations as are necessary to the acquisition of a thorough anatomical knowledge.

I need not repeat that it relates to those parts so interesting as concerns the theory of cerebral localizations, namely, the *thalami optici*, the *caudated ganglion*, the *lenticular ganglion*, and the *internal capsule*. Such are the various constituents which united form that which is called the *central system*, in distinction from the *cortical system*.

Bring to mind how the crura cerebri, rounded at the point where they border the thalami optici, flatten after having passed it, internally and externally spreading forward and backward like a fan. Upon that fan—allow me to continue the simile—the ganglia of the gray substance are arranged as follows: the *thalami optici* within and posteriorly; within, but before and above, the *caudated ganglion*; outside of the fan, and below the thalami optici and caudated ganglion, is situated the *lenticular ganglion*, which extends nearly as far forward as the head of the corpus striatum, and backward nearly as far as the posterior extremity of the thalami optici.

I only wish to indicate, *en passant*, the forms and principal relations of the gray ganglia which I have enumerated.

1st. The *thalamus opticus* has a flattened, ovoid appearance. The superior face looks upon the lateral ventricle, and the inferior, which is also the internal, upon the middle ventricle. On dissection it is with difficulty separated, on account of its numerous and close connections with contiguous parts.

2d. The *caudated ganglion* has the form of a comma — or of a pyramid — the large end of which is directed forward and inward, the small end upward and outward. Its superior face protrudes into the ventricle; the so-called internal face is mostly in contact with the superior portion of the internal capsule. This ganglion is very easily detached in dissections, but in order to isolate it, the numerous fasciculi which it receives from the internal capsule must be broken.

3d. The *lenticular ganglion*, although all its surface is covered, can easily and without much art be isolated from the neighboring parts. Its general form is ovoid, with an anterior and a posterior extremity. There can be distinguished in it two parts: (*a*) The anterior third, more obtuse, and composed of a uniform mass of gray substance, is, at its very anterior extremity, confounded with the intraventricular nucleus of the corpus striatum. (*b*) The second portion, the posterior two-thirds of the lenticular ganglion, is flattened from above downward in such wise as to offer an angle turned inward towards the internal capsule. The internal and superior face is intimately united to the internal capsule, and the inferior face is parallel with the base of the brain. The external face is in *rapport* with the external capsule, and its intermediate with the front wall of the island of Reil. The island lies close to it in its entire extent. An interesting preparation consists in carefully removing successively the gray substance of the convolutions of the island, the anterior wall, and the external capsule, which lays bare the external face of the lenticular ganglion.

In hardened specimens the separation between the external face of the lenticular ganglion and the external capsule is effected without art and with the utmost ease. This is because there are no medullary fasciculi — and you see that there are no vessels—which bind the external capsule to the third segment of the lenticular ganglion.

From the connections which we have outlined it might be said that the three ganglia or gray central masses—thalamus opticus, caudated ganglion, and lenticular ganglion—are in some sense, as Foville has said, appendices to the internal capsule, like cotyledonal prolongations of the crura cerebri.

On the side of the ventricles the thalami optici and the caudated ganglia are isolated ; the lenticular ganglion is also isolated, virtually, at least, on the side of the island. These gray ganglia, then, form a distinct system from the other parts of the brain, as well by their connections as by their mode of vascularization.

Vertical sections will enable you to easily understand the relations of the central parts. I will not at this point dwell upon the structural details of the different ganglia, but will return to them as occasion requires. Some examination and idea of the construction of the internal capsule, however, is indispensable.

The *internal capsule*, in part at least, is the prolongation, not of the entire crus cerebri, but of the *foot* or *crusta*, the *inferior part* only. The *tegmentum* or *superior part*, which is separated from the foot by the *locus niger*, enters into relations especially with the tubercula quadrigemina and the thalami optici ; it takes no direct part in the formation of the internal capsule.

An old opinion held the internal capsule as a complete and immediate emanation from the foot of the diverging fibres. This is an error which Luys and Kölliker have corrected. These authors have, in fact, demonstrated that the fibres coming from the peduncle stop by the way to enter various ganglia. I think, however, they have gone too far, in holding that the internal capsule is entirely formed, 1st, of diverging

5

fibres which terminate in the ganglia ; 2d, of fibres which leave the ganglia and become diverging fibres.

From very delicate anatomical observations, Meynert, Henle, and Broadbent have expressed the opinion that there exists a third order of fibres which communicates directly from the foot of the peduncle to the gray cortex.

The verification of the existence of these last fasciculi depends, as you will see, upon certain pathological proofs. I will cite, among others, some cases of descending degenerations observed by Vulpian and myself. In the cases referred to, destruction and yellow spots had largely invaded the median convolutions, without concomitant alterations of the corpora striata, and had produced progressive degeneration, which could be followed across the isthmus and to the lower region of the spinal cord. We are indebted to Gudden for a series of experiments which I will later have occasion to notice, and the results of which have the same bearing.

Henle[1] goes too far, perhaps, when he writes in his description of the nervous system that the internal capsule is composed *entirely* of the fibres from the foot of the peduncle. Certainly—and we will have occasion to return to this subject—both pathological and experimental facts in favor of the existence of these fibres are numerous and important, and the facts permit a belief (we will further on see the demonstration), that among the direct fibres some (the anterior) are centrifugal and connected with movements of the limbs, while others (the posterior) are centripetal and connected with the transmission of sensorial impressions (Fig. 18).

To sum up, the *internal capsule*, according to modern researches,[2] is composed as follows :

1st. By the *direct peduncular fasciculi*, which traverse the capsule without entering the ganglia.

2d. By the *indirect peduncular fasciculi.* Of these some are sent to the corpora striata, which they approach by the inferior face ; others go to the lenticular ganglia, which they

[1] Henle.—Nervenlehre, p. 261.
[2] Huguenin.—Allg. Patholog. der Krankh. des Nervensystems; Zurich, 1873, p. 94, Fig. 70; p. 85, Fig. 63; p. 119, Fig. 82; p. 127.

penetrate by its first segment. Very numerous in this segment, they become less and less in the second and third seg-

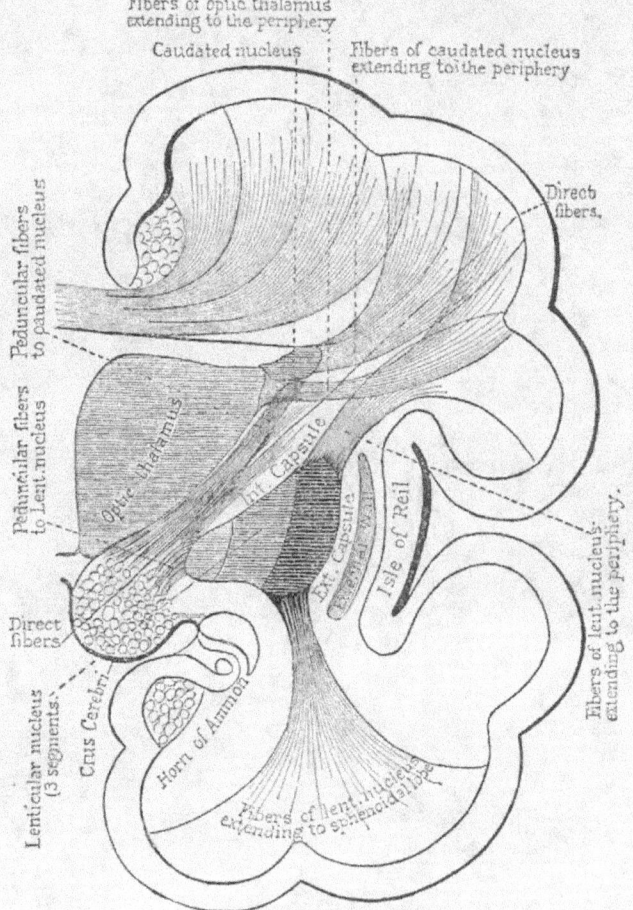

FIG. 18.—Scheme illustrative of the different orders of peduncular fibres.—*Huguenin.*

ments, and to that unequal distribution is due the difference in color of the three segments of the lenticular ganglion.

There is no question as to whether the fibres from the foot of the peduncle go to the thalami optici; the thalami optici receive no other fasciculi from the cerebral peduncles except those from the *tegmentum*.

To the fasciculi which go from the *foot* of the peduncle to

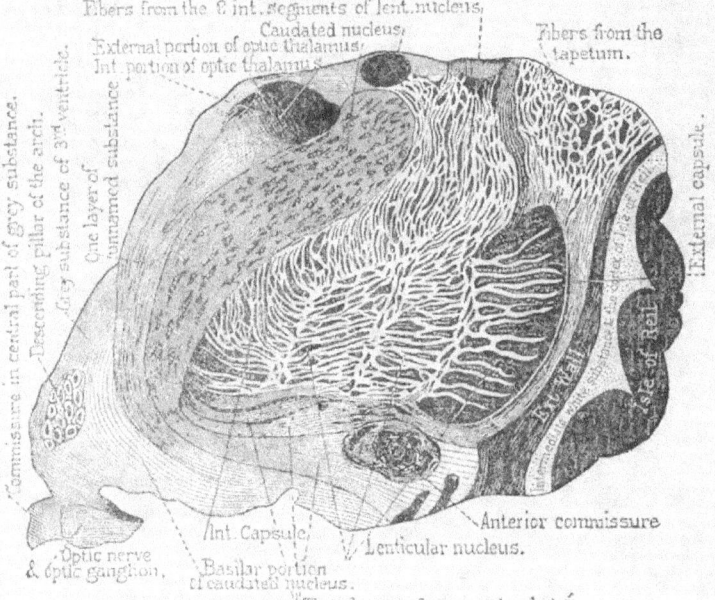

Fig. 19.—Section of lenticular ganglion and its surroundings.—(*Meynert.*)

the gray central ganglia are added, in the superior part of the internal capsule, fasciculi which originate in the gray ganglia, and go towards forming the diverging fibres that run to the gray layer of the cortex. These fasciculi bear the name of radiating fasciculi (*Stabkranzbündel*). There can be distinguished, 1st, the diverging fasciculi of the corpora striata ; 2d, the radiating fasciculi of the thalami optici ; 3d, the radiating fasciculi issuing from the lenticular ganglion, which come principally from the superior border of the second and third segments.

It follows from this exhibit that four orders of fasciculi enter into the composition of the diverging fibres, and so attach the internal capsule to the cortex of the convolution.

They are : 1st, the radiating fasciculi of the thalami optici ; 2d, those of the corpora striata ; 3d, those of the lenticular ganglion—these various fasciculi attach the gray central ganglia to the cortex ; 4th, the direct fasciculi which go from the foot of the peduncle to the gray cortex without stopping in the gray central ganglia.

In the internal capsule itself, and also in the foot of the diverging fibres, one can recognize these various modes of origin by submitting thin slices, properly hardened, to a low power of the microscope ; to be sure, the research is not exempt from difficulty. A little above that point, however, all the fasciculi intermix in the most varied manner, either among themselves, or it may be with the commissural fibres, in such manner as to form an inextricable net-work, called the central white substance. We will soon render an exact account of the interest pertaining to this arrangement.

EIGHTH AND NINTH LECTURES.

CENTRAL ARTERIES.—ISOLATED LESIONS OF THE GRAY GANGLIA.

Summary:—Origin of the Arterial System of the Central Ganglionic Masses.—Unequal Participation of the Main Arteries of the Brain Constituting this System.—Description of the Striated Arteries; Internal Striated Arteries; External Striated Arteries (Lenticulo-Striated, Lenticulo-Optic).—Terminal Arteries.—Consequences of Obliterations of Central Arteries Emanating from the Sylvian Artery.—Softening of the Optico-Striated Bodies.—Intra-Encephalic Hemorrhage.—Regional Diagnosis.—Isolated Lesions of the Gray Ganglia without Participation of the Internal Capsule.—Cerebral Hemiplegia, Central and Cortical.—Lesions of the Internal Capsule.—Variations of Symptoms according to the Spot in the Internal Capsule Occupied by the Lesions.—New Anatomical Considerations: Peduncular Fibres going Directly to the Cortical Substance of the Occipital Lobe; their Rôle Relative to Sensibility.—Proofs Furnished, 1st, by Lesions of the Posterior Lenticulo-Optic Regions of the Internal Capsule (Hemi-Anæsthesia Cerebral); 2d, by Experimentation.

GENTLEMEN:

I. You remember that the three great arteries of the brain take an unequal part in forming the arterial *system of the central ganglionic masses*.

A.—(*a.*) Thus, the *Sylvian artery* very greatly predominates. It furnishes: 1st, in great part, the *caudated ganglion ;* 2d, the entire lenticular ganglion ; 3d, a portion of the *thalamus opticus ;* 4th, the whole extent of the *internal capsule.*

(*b.*) The *anterior cerebral artery* has, on the contrary, very modest attributes. It arterializes only the head of the caudated ganglion, and even in this its participation is not constant.

(*c.*) As for the posterior cerebral artery, its rôle is more important and tolerably characteristic. That artery, which is extensively distributed (as it sends branches to the choroid plexuses, to the ventricular walls, etc.), furnishes the following regions of the central masses: 1st, the external and posterior part of the thalami optici; 2d, the tubercula quadrigemina; 3d, the superior portions of the crura cerebri.

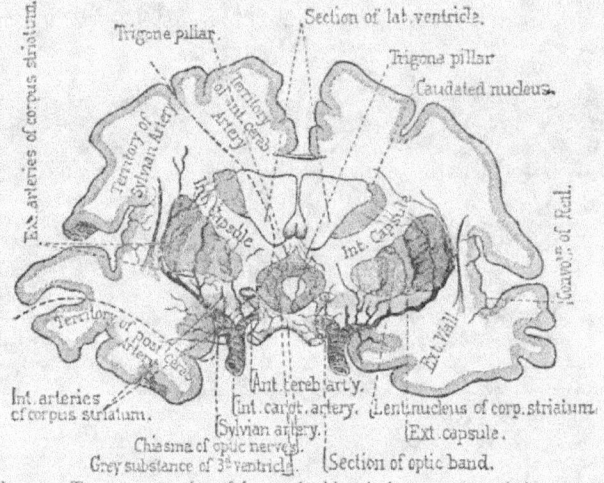

FIG. 20.—Transverse section of the cerebral hemispheres, one centimètre posterior to the optic chiasma. Arteries of the corpora striata.—(*Duret.*) Vascular territories indicated by dotted lines.

The plates (Figs. 20 and 21), on which the vascular territories are separated by dotted lines, will make the details clearer.

The description of the *striated arteries* alone requires some explanation. With this you will possess, in brief, all that is necessary to a knowledge of the central arteries, whether they come from the anterior or the posterior cerebral arteries.

Emanating from the superior border of the Sylvian artery, the striated arteries enter the apertures of the anterior perforated space, where they soon disappear from sight. But a very simple preparation renders it possible to follow them in the first part of their intracerebral course. I solicit attention to the following description, because that, in order to understand some important facts, it is indispensable to know the theory of common cerebral hemorrhage.

That exposition consists in destroying successively the gray cortex of the island of Reil, the subjacent white substance, the anterior wall, and finally the internal capsule.

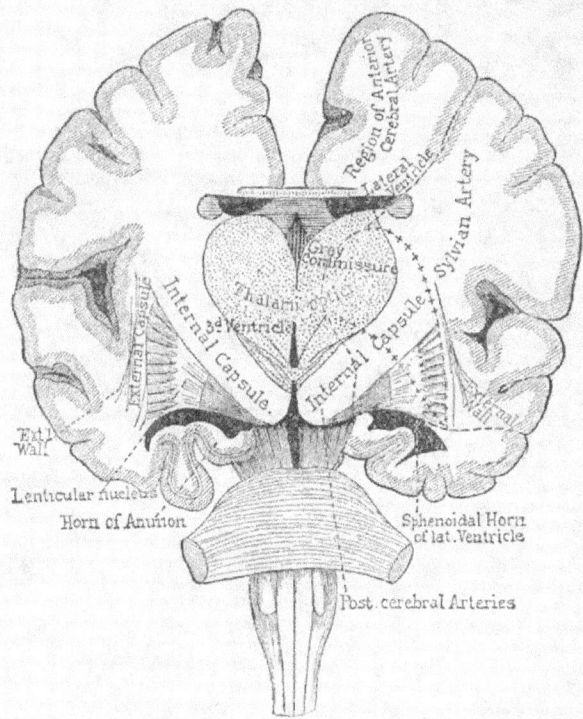

FIG. 21.—Vertico-transverse section of the human brain, posterior to the tubercula mammillaria and anterior to the peduncles. Vascular territories indicated by dotted lines.

Thus the entire external surface of the lenticular ganglion is laid bare. If the preparation has been somewhat carefully made, upon a well-injected brain—and the preparation is easily made, because, in its anterior part at least, the lenticular ganglion is as it were naturally detached from the internal capsule—one can follow the first part of the distribution of the principal striated arteries. By this artifice it is seen that they spread like a fan at the surface of the gray ganglia. But at a short distance from their origin they bury themselves in the substance of the third segment, where they disappear.

Now, it is upon the transverse sections that one must follow the ulterior distribution of the striated arteries.

A first section, made behind the chiasma (Fig. 20), shows only the caudated and lenticular ganglia, the thalami optici being more posterior. Upon that section are found the deepest tracts of the arteries which we have just had under observation. Besides these, other and smaller arterioles may be discovered on the external surface of the lenticular ganglia, and which may be termed *internal;* after detaching themselves from the Sylvian trunk, they rise nearly perpendicularly into the first two segments of the lenticular ganglion and the adjoining parts of the internal capsule.

Of still greater interest are the *external striated arteries*, those which, in the first part of their course, run over the external face of the lenticular ganglia. They should be divided into two groups: the first group is anterior, and the arteries of which it is composed are the *lenticulo-striated arteries;* the second group is posterior, and the arteries which constitute it are the *lenticulo-optic arteries.*

One of the arteries in the anterior group is especially important on account of its size and its predominant rôle in intra-encephalic hemorrhage; it could be appropriately called the *artery of cerebral hemorrhage.* After having entered the third segment it traverses the superior portion of the internal capsule, then enters the body of the caudated ganglion. It then continues from behind forward to the most anterior part of that ganglion.

The distribution of this striated artery, as well as that of the lenticulo-striated arteries, should be studied from sections made anterior to the one which has thus far served us.

The *lenticulo-optic arteries* are after the same model, only after having traversed the most posterior part of the internal capsule, they encounter the external and anterior part of the thalamus opticus, over which they spread.

I would remind you that we are dealing with *terminal arteries*, and that if the injections are too strongly pressed they will produce little ruptures upon different points of the vascular tract, thus imitating in locality, as well as in form, the centres of hemorrhage which are produced pathologically.

About the branches of the *anterior cerebral artery*, we have nothing especial to say, except that they do not constantly exist, and that they give place to very circumscribed hemorrhages, though really grave, inasmuch as they often open into the ventricles.

As for the *posterior cerebral artery*, I repeat that it merits by itself more minute attention. I only wish to notice here the arteries which it sends to the thalami optici.

These arteries are of two orders : 1st, the *posterior internal optic artery*, arising from the posterior cerebral near its origin at the basilar trunk, and which furnishes the internal face of the thalamus opticus, and is capable in its ulterior tracts of occasioning hemorrhages, of small extent to be sure, but serious, as being often followed by ventricular inundation ; 2d, the *posterior external optic artery*, which comes from the posterior cerebral after it has passed around the crus cerebri, and in which it ascends obliquely before entering the posterior part of the thalamus opticus. The rupture of this vessel produces hemorrhage which often breaks into the body of the crura cerebri. This artery deserves your close attention, for, as you will see later, lesions within its territory produce a train of symptoms altogether peculiar to themselves.

II. In journeying along we have gathered facts in the highest degree interesting for the theory of cerebral pathological localizations, and we will now examine these facts more closely, commencing with those which concern the central ganglionic masses.

A. (*a.*) The entire system of the central arteries emanating from the Sylvian, may be obliterated in consequence of a thrombus or an embolus of the principal arterial trunk. Then follows softening of nearly the entire mass of the gray ganglia, the district corresponding to the anterior cerebral and the *posterior optic* arteries alone being spared. Here is a very concise *localization*, generally of an extreme gravity, and which embraces, clinically speaking, all the pathology of. the ganglionic centres. The symptoms which belong to a softening of the entire *optico-striated bodies* (the entire central masses are sometimes so called) are none other than common *cerebral hemiplegia accompanied with cerebral hemi-anæsthesia*.

(*b.*) Analysis may be brought to bear on this complex whole. We must not believe, however, that we are at present able to recognize the special symptoms which belong to the destruction of the thalami optici, the caudated ganglia, or the lenticular ganglia, and still less to the various segments.

(*c.*) It is possible, however, by reason of the arterial distribution which we have described, that the anatomical locality may betray itself by special symptoms, thus affording a *regional diagnosis*. This is realized when the softening affects all, or nearly all, of the territory of the lenticulo-striated arteries, or that of the lenticulo-optic arteries. The two different events differ in their symptoms ; the symptoms of hemianæsthesia are present when the field of the lenticulo-optic arteries is invaded, and absent when the lenticulo-striated arteries are the ones involved.

B. That which has been said relative to ischæmic softening is also applicable to *intra-encephalic hemorrhage*. This, you know, is frequent, and especially in these regions ; the striated arteries are, indeed, very prone to a special form of arterial sclerosis which produces *miliary aneurisms*. One often extracts from a recent hemorrhagic centre a striate or an optic artery, the prolongations of which have small aneurisms.[1]

Contrary to current opinion, sanguineous effusion generally occurs (as Gendrin has long since recognized[2]), in such cases, not at first in the body of the corpus striatum itself, but outside of it—to be more exact, in contact with the external surface of the lenticular ganglion, between that and

[1] See plate V. of *Archives de physiologie*, 1868.
[2] A. N. Gendrin, *Traité philosophique de médecine pratique*, t. I., 1838. See page 443, Nos. 789, 796 ; p. 465, Nos. 808, 809, 810 ; and page 478, No. 830.

the *external capsule*, which becomes detached. Thus are produced those flat centres which upon transverse sections appear like narrow linear lacunæ, nearly vertical, and parallel to the gray ganglion of the front wall (Fig. 22). When the sanguineous effusion is abundant the hemorrhagic centre extends, especially transversely, and on account of the greater resistance of the cranial walls and the wall of the island, the central masses, enucleated so to speak, are crowded back *en bloc* towards the ventricular cavity (Fig. 22).

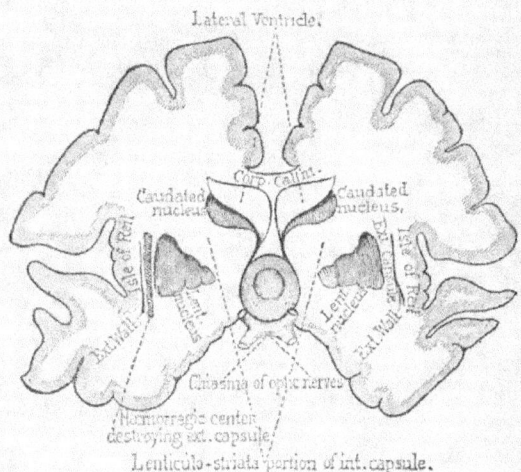

FIG. 22.—Extra-lenticular hemorrhagic centre, posterior to the optic chiasma. (*No hemianæsthesia.*)

I have given very ordinary cases, but it may happen also that extravasation coming from the extremities of the terminal arteries will occur in the body even of either the corpus striatum or of the thalamus opticus.

Be that as it may, the only clinical localization possible in these cases is, as in case of softening, those which correspond to the lenticulo-striated or the lenticulo-optic domains.

The symptoms of hemorrhage are at present more difficult of interpretation or of exact localizing than are those of softening. Uninformed, one would be liable to attribute certain symptoms to the *destruction* of a part which really was only the result of a neighboring accident. I allude to compression, which, during effusion, however slight it may be, never fails to somewhat affect the adjacent parts This is a point to which I will shortly return.

III. The definitely acquired facts relative to *regional diagnosis* concerning the various parts which enter into the composition of the central ganglionic masses of the brain can be reduced to a very small number of propositions.

1st. Regarding lesions confined to any one of the gray central ganglia, and *where the internal capsule is not involved*, we are not at present able, from clinical examination, to recognize any special characters.

(*a.*) Thus it is impossible to distinguish, during life, a lesion limited to the lenticular ganglion from one confined to the caudated ganglion, and lesions of the thalamus opticus (though upon this last point there is reason perhaps for some reserve) generally confound themselves clinically with those produced in the two compartments of the corpus striatum.

The symptoms which accompany lesions limited to the gray central ganglia are those of *common cerebral hemiplegia*. That form of cerebral hemiplegia may be called *central*, to distinguish it from motor paralysis, which sometimes results from superficial lesions, and which in distinction I will call *cortical cerebral hemiplegia*.

(*b.*) Paralysis, dependent upon lesions of the gray central ganglia, is generally of motion only; disturbances of sensation such as belong to *cerebral hemianæsthesia* are, however, sometimes added, under special circumstances to which we will shortly give attention.

(*c.*) Hemiplegia, dependent upon alterations confined to the gray ganglia, is generally transitory, passing, lightly marked not indelible, and in any case is at first comparatively benign. It is understood that in formulating this proposition I remove all complications capable of greatly modifying the picture; such, for example, would be the eruption of a hemorrhage, however small, into a ventricular cavity.

Grave symptoms, such as *early contractions*, or *epileptiform convulsions*, almost necessarily ensue in such cases, and more or less rapid death is generally the necessary consequence of such complication.

The relative benignity of lesions limited to the gray ganglia arises in part, doubtless, from the fact that these ganglia are scarcely ever affected in their totality. Thus the caudated ganglion, for example (and the fact is explained by the method in which the vessels going to it are distributed), is never destroyed in its entire extent, at least by itself, that is to say, without the participation of the *internal capsule* or other gray ganglia. On the other hand, the transitory character of a paralysis resulting from partial lesion of the central ganglionic masses may indicate, as we will see, a sort of *functional supplement* established between the various parts of the caudated ganglion, or between the caudated ganglion and the various segments of the lenticular ganglion.

2d. Then, again, lesions of the *internal capsule*, even when strictly limited to the white tract, in no degree including the substance of the gray ganglia—these lesions, I say, generally produce common cerebral hemiplegia of a very marked and more or less persisting form. Thus, even when very circumscribed (principally when they are situated low down at the side of the peduncle), these lesions produce a motor paralysis almost necessarily accompanied by *late contractions ;* a symptom of bad augury in these troubles, because as a rule it announces that the paralysis will resist all therapeutical means.

3d. It is proper to establish here an important distinction. We have already said that the symptoms differ remarkably according to the portion of the internal capsule affected by the lesion.

If it occupies any part of the *anterior two-thirds of the capsule*, the region where the white tract separates the anterior extremity of the lenticular ganglion from the head of the caudated ganglion, and which belong, as you know, to the field of the lenticulo-striated artery, the *paralysis* will be exclusively that of *motion ;* there will be no durable trouble of sensation.

On the contrary, if the lesion having invaded the domain of the lenticulo-optic arteries should extend to the posterior third of the capsule, in that region where it passes between the posterior extremity of the lenticular ganglion and the thalamus opticus, the presence of cerebral hemianæsthesia would be almost certain. Most frequently the lesion extends

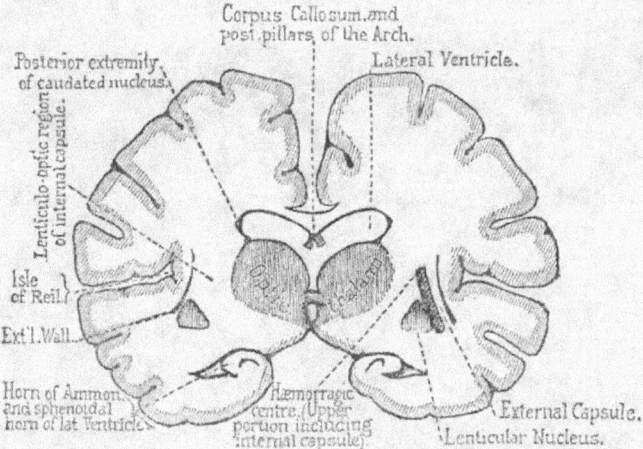

FIG. 23.—Extra-lenticular hemorrhagic centre on a plane with the posterior portion of the thalamus opticus. (*Cerebral hemianæsthesia.*)

to several parts, and paralysis of sensation will be accompanied with a more or less marked motor hemiplegia. But it may happen that cerebral hemianæsthesia will occur alone, at least as a permanent phenomenon, in those cases, for example, where the most distant parts, the most posterior portion of the internal capsule would alone be definitely altered (Fig. 23).

In the preceding exposé I have purposely alluded only to truly *destructive lesions* of the internal capsule, to those which, either by lacerations or necrosis, produce an irreparable loss of substance. It is necessary, however, to distinguish those cases where the internal capsule is not directly involved, but affected by proximity to a neighboring phenomenon, that is, the consequence of a lesion limited to the

gray ganglia which surround the capsules.   Thus the disten-
tion of one of these ganglia, in case of interstitial hemorrhage, might compress the nerve-fibres that compose the internal capsule and so suspend their functions.   But as the
nerve-fibres in such cases are only compromised and not destroyed, the paralytic phenomena resulting from that compression (excepting cases of tumor) would always be temporary.

The combination which I have brought to your notice is
frequently met in the clinic of intracerebral hemorrhage ; it
makes a somewhat complicated condition, and one in which
the interpretation of symptoms might be rendered difficult.
In this way, if one is not well forewarned of the difficulties,

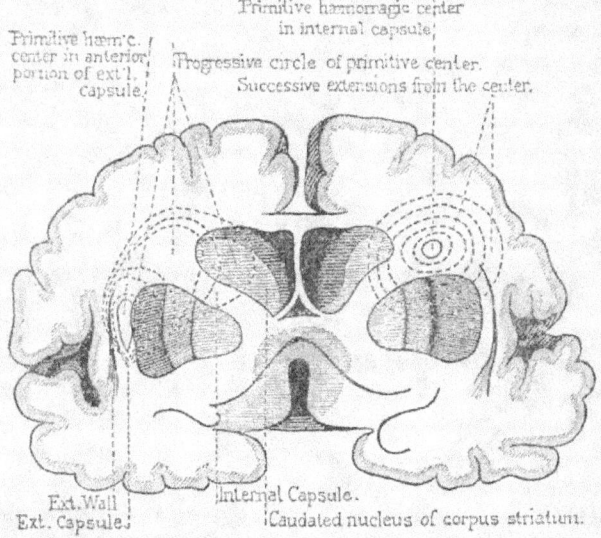

Fig. 24.—Human brain. Section through the *anterior* portion of the internal
capsule, showing the location, mode of formation, and extension of hemorrhages at
the anterior portion of the internal capsule.   (*Hemiplegias.*)

they would be tempted (and the error has often been com-
mitted) to attribute certain symptoms to destruction of some
one of the gray ganglia, as to the thalamus opticus, or the

corpus striatum, which were only the result of a neighboring accident and the incidental compression of the internal capsule.

The subject is worth further explanations.

Let us suppose the recent formation of a hemorrhagic centre in the *lieu d'élection*. The blood would then be extravasated outside of the lenticular ganglion, virtually into the space of which we have already spoken ; and the third segment of the lenticular ganglion, otherwise called the *putamen*, would generally be in part torn away. I have told you that under such circumstances the external wall of the extravasated spot, including the convolutions of the island of Reil, the anterior wall, and the internal capsule, would resist the pressure of the extravasated blood, while the gray ganglia are generally crowded in their entirety towards the ventricular cavities. It is clear that the substance of the internal capsule would necessarily be more or less forcibly compressed by such a change (Fig. 24). Respecting the symptoms produced, two conditions might ensue.

Sometimes the extravasated centre is restricted to those portions of the lenticular ganglion which correspond to the anterior half or two-thirds of that body ; that is, to the domain of the lenticulo-striated artery. In consequence, *the anterior part of the internal capsule* would be immediately affected by compression. The effect would be exclusively a motor hemiplegia of the opposite side of the body (Fig. 22). Sometimes, generally extending from before backward, the extravasation would crowd to the most posterior parts of the lenticular ganglion ; pressure would then be made upon *the posterior part of the internal capsule*, and symptoms of cerebral hemianæsthesia would follow those of motor hemiplegia.

Figures 24 and 25 will enable you to easily recognize the precise locality, and the mode of formation and extension of the various centres of central hemorrhage (see also Fig. 23).

One word more upon the interpretation of these facts. After having recognized during life the following symptoms ; motor hemiplegia with hemianæsthesia, and at *post-mortem* the existence of a spot involving the lenticular ganglion,

6

would you be led to conclude from the close relation of these
two orders of facts that the lenticular ganglion controlled both
sensation and voluntary motion of the opposite side ?

Such conclusion would not be very legitimate, for, had the
patient survived, and the extravasation absorbed and left as
a representative only a yellow linear cicatrix, the hemianæsthesia, and even the motor paralysis, notwithstanding partial
destruction of the lenticular ganglion, would doubtless have
disappeared, leaving no traces.

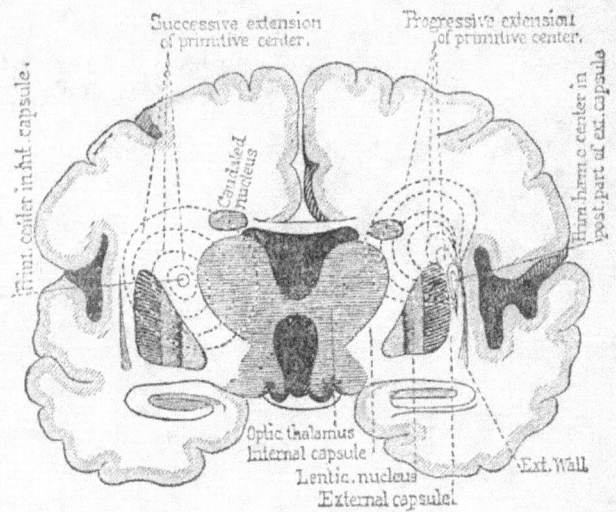

FIG. 25.—Human brain. Section through the *posterior* portion of the internal
capsule, showing location, mode of formation and extension of hemorrhages at the
posterior portion of the internal capsule. (*Hemianæsthesia.*)

That which has been said respecting hemorrhages of the
lenticular ganglion applies equally to hemorrhages which occur in the posterior portion of the bodies of the thalami optici. These hemorrhages result from a rupture of the external
anterior optic, or lenticulo-optic artery. They are generally
indicated by a more or less marked hemiplegia, and nearly
always also by a more or less complete hemianæsthesia, provided the hemorrhage be sufficiently extensive. Should it

be at once concluded (as so many authors have said and still repeat) that the thalami optici are the seat of *common sensation?* Incontestably, no ; besides, it would be easy to cite numbers of facts where a hemorrhagic lesion of the posterior tract of the thalamus opticus produced, in the first phase of the malady (that is to say, when conditions of pressure existed), sensitive and sensorial disturbances, which disturbances ceased in the later stage, that is, from the date where reabsorption removed the pressure from the posterior or lenticulo-optic region of the internal capsule.

It would be superfluous to continue. I think I have sufficiently demonstrated that in regional diagnosis, as concerns the various parts of the central masses of the brain, it is the participation or the non-participation of the anterior or posterior regions of the internal capsule which determines the situation.

IV. The propositions which I have offered possess a practical interest which will not escape your attention. Hitherto they have been presented in the form of a *postulate.* It is now proper to establish them by demonstration ; or, in other terms, to give you that proof which will serve to insure them a permanent place in the records of human pathology.

We ought also to give, as far as we can, the theory of the facts concerned ; that is, we should enter as far as possible into the anatomical and pathological reasons. To accomplish this, we are obliged to return once more to the normal anatomy of the brain, in order to complete in some respects the ideas already acquired.

In the preceding *exposé,* the predominant rôle in the pathological anatomy of the central masses which is sustained by the two main departments of the internal capsule, has been shown, together with the proof, and they justify the descriptions which we have made concerning the anatomical constitution of the grand tract. Now, it is necessary to go a little further, and seek for that which is peculiar to the anterior or lenticulo-striated region of the capsule, in distinction from that which is peculiar to the posterior, or lenticulo-optic region, where lesions produce only symptoms of *cerebral hemi-anæsthesia*. We will commence with the last.

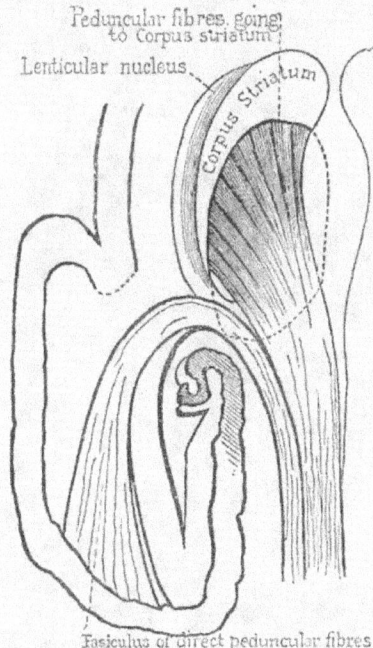

Peduncular fibres going to Corpus striatum

Lenticular nucleus.

Corpus Striatum

Fasiculus of direct peduncular fibres going to cortical substance of occip.¹ lobe.

FIG. 26.—Scheme of direct and indirect peduncular fibres.—(*Huguenin.*)

A. The recent anatomical researches of Meynert have furnished us in this respect with very important information. They have been given in detail in a work of one of his auditors, Huguenin, Professor at Zurich.[1] They consist of dissections and also in comparisons of thin slices, hardened, and examined by transmitted light.

The brain being placed upon its base, the lateral ventricles are opened in such manner as to lay bare the superior face of the central masses—those which are contiguous to the various parts of the isthmus; after that, by minute dissection, are successively removed: 1st, *tegmentum*, or upper part of the peduncle; 2d, the tubercula quadrigemina; 3d, the entire thalami optici.

This being done, the inferior parts of the peduncle (*pes, crusta*) are brought to view, and higher up (in the region of the internal capsule), the fasciculi of peduncular fibres running to the caudated ganglion. The fibres belonging to the internal capsule, which go to the lenticular ganglion, occupy a plane situated beneath and external to the preceding fasciculi.

---

[1] Allgem. Path. der Krankh., etc., p. 119, Fig. 82, Zurich, 1873.

Attentively observing the internal and posterior parts of the diverging fibres thus exposed, there is to be discovered a fasciculus, detached as it were from the main body, and which, without entering the substance of the gray ganglia, turns backward as soon as it reaches the inferior border of the lenticular ganglion (Fig. 26).

That, you see, is a direct fasciculus, since the fibres of which it is composed enter the diverging fibres without stopping in the gray substance of the central masses; it is, moreover, as the description shows, a separate fasciculus.

What is the destination of these nerve-fibres? With man it is nearly impossible to say; but in some monkeys, according to Meynert, their course can be easily followed into the body of the white substance of the occipital lobe, just outside the posterior cornu of the lateral ventricle (*cornu posterius, ventriculi lateralis*). They finally terminate in the body of the gray cortical substance of the occipital lobe.

B. Does there exist any anatomical reason for supposing that the fasciculus in question is really composed of centripetal fibres, having as a function the transmission of sensitive impressions to the surface of the posterior regions of the brain? Meynert so thinks, and for the reason that (according to him) these fibres, by comparing thin slices, can be followed down the length of the cerebral peduncle to the protuberance (foot, inferior part); in the peduncle they occupy the most external part. Reaching the protuberance, they go to the posterior part of the pyramidal fasciculus, and maintain very nearly the same location in the anterior pyramid to the point of decussation. There (contrary to that which occurs with the most internal fasciculi of the pyramid, which pass into the lateral columns of the spinal cord) they decussate, and then join the posterior spinal fasciculi. I am not able to guarantee the entire authenticity of the last part of the tract assigned by Meynert to the fibres which compose the most posterior portion of the internal capsule.

Such is at present the share of normal anatomy, and it affords an independent illumination of our subject. But however important this aid, it would, without pathological anatomy and experimentation, be entirely insufficient to solve the problem ; and once more we repeat that physiology and pathology cannot be deduced from an unassisted contemplation of pure anatomical facts.

C. We are now at the proper point to introduce clinical and anatomico-pathological proofs. At the present time they are abundant. It will suffice to note the observations of Ludwig Türck, the pioneer in this road,[1] those of his compatriot Rosenthal,[2] those which I have collected at the Salpêtrière, and finally those which have been gathered by Veyssière and Rendu, the first in his inaugural thesis,[3] the second in his thesis for *agrégation*.[4]

The comparison of these observations gives the following uniform results : 1st, that lesions confined to the posterior lenticulo-optic region of the internal capsule necessarily result in that form of hemianæsthesia which I call cerebral, and in which sensations controlled by the cerebral nerves, that is, the optic and olfactory nerves, are so affected as to faithfully reproduce the characteristics of hysterical hemianæsthesia ; 2d, that on the contrary, in all cases where the lesions involve only that part of the capsule which lies between the lenticular ganglion and the head of the caudated ganglion, anæsthesia is absent.

These contributions of pathological anatomy and clinic are by themselves of incontestable and prime importance ; but combined with the testimony of pure anatomy, they assume a standard value.

That is not all ; experimentation has in turn brought its share of facts, which also repeat the same story.

Under the guidance of pathological knowledge, experimentation has corrected itself. It had previously been sup-

---

[1] Türck, see Charcot.—Lectures upon Maladies of the Nervous System, t. I., 2d ed., p. 315.

[2] Rosenthal, Klinik der Nervenkrankheiten, 2d Aufl., Stuttgart, 1875.

[3] R. Veyssière, Recherches clniques et expérimentales sur l'hémianesthésie de cause cérébrale. Thèse de Paris, 1874.

[4] H. Rendu, Des anesthésies spontanées. Thèse d'agrégation, Paris, 1875, pp. 27 and 95.

posed that the centre of sensitive impressions was not in the brain proper, nor in the thalami optici, but lower down, in the protuberance, or perhaps in the crura cerebri.

Pathology controverted that assertion, in showing that a lesion situated above those points, in certain regions of the brain itself, was quite sufficient to invariably produce a total hemianæsthesia. Recent experimental researches made by Duret and Veyssière, in the laboratory of Vulpian, have given results also in conformity with pathological teaching.

An ingenious instrument, consisting of a trocar from which at a desired moment escapes a spring, is introduced through the cranial

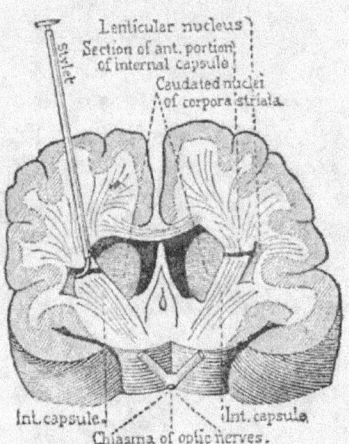

Fig. 27.—Transverse section of a dog's brain, five millimètres anterior to the optic chiasma.

wall into the central masses, to a depth and in a direction calculated through previous experiments. Thus, with a little experience, either of the two portions of the internal capsule can by itself be injured.

If in these experiments the lesion reaches the posterior capsule, hemianæsthesia of the opposite side of the body certainly ensues; generally there is associated with it a certain degree of motor paralysis; this (motor paralysis), on the contrary, occurs unaccompanied with anæsthesia whenever the lesion is confined to any point of the anterior two-thirds, leaving the posterior third of the internal capsule untouched. (Figs. 27 and 28.)

Such in brief are the substantial results of these experiments.

After the foregoing, you will see that everything concurs to establish the existence of direct fasciculi of centripetal nerve-fibres in the posterior part of the internal capsule, having for function the conduction of sensitive impressions coming from the opposite side of the body towards the centre.

Emanating from the foot of the central peduncle, these fasciculi, as they leave the capsule, run directly towards the formation of the diverging fibres, without communicating with the gray ganglia of the central masses. Near their origin, that is, at the inferior part of the capsule, these fasciculi, pressed into a narrow space, might be affected in great num-

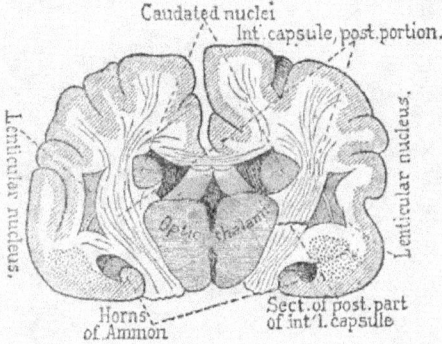

FIG. 28.—Transverse section of a dog's brain, on a plane with the tubercula mammillaria.—(*Carville and Duret.*)

bers by a single stroke, by a very minute lesion, and be followed by very marked anæsthesia. It can be understood, on the other hand, that higher up, on a level with the foot of the diverging fibres, a lesion of the same extent would, by reason of the divergence of the fibres, produce much less marked effects. This is, in fact, the case. There exist many examples of well-marked hemianæsthesia in connection with slight lesions of the foot of the diverging fibres.

It should now be determined if lesions extended to the occipital lobes, and especially to their gray cortex, produce crossed hemianæsthesia. Unhappily the facts which can be cited in that regard are not sufficiently explicit, and the question must remain in suspense until more ample information is obtained.[1] However that may be, it is now recognized

---

[1] In the observations which I have collected of superficial softenings of the occipital lobe, there were frequent hyperæsthesias, painful sensations of all sorts in the opposite limbs, hallucinations of vision, etc., as well as hemianæsthesia or amblyopia.

that the fasciculi which compose the posterior part of the internal capsule, and their direct emanations, cannot be considered as a centre of sensitive and sensorial impressions. These fasciculi can only represent a highway, a cross-road, where the centripetal fibres of which it is composed are all represented before diverging to the superficial parts of the brain.

TENTH LECTURE.

CEREBRAL HEMIANÆSTHESIA (CONTINUED).—CROSSED AMBLYOPIA.—LATERAL HEMIOPIA.

Summary :—Resume of the Characters of Cerebral Hemianæsthesia.—Its Resemblance to Hysterical Hemianæsthesia.—Anæsthesia Involves General Sensibility in its Various Forms, and also the Special Senses.—Hysterical Amblyopia.—Ophthalmoscopic Examination.—Concerning Functions.—Diminution of Visual Acuteness.—Concentric and General Contraction of the Field of Vision, etc.—Crossed Amblyopia with Hemianæsthesia from Cerebral Causes.—Symptoms.—Lesions of the Cerebral Hemispheres which Produce Hemianæsthesia Produce also Crossed Amblyopia and not Lateral Hemiopia.—Hemiopia.—Hypothesis of Semidecussation.—Unilateral Homologous Hemiopia.—Varieties of Hemiopia.

GENTLEMEN :

In the last lecture I attempted to prove that a peculiar form of hemianæsthesia is a necessary consequence of lesions in the posterior regions of the internal capsule, or of its emanations in the diverging fibres, no matter whether these lesions be destructive, compressive, or suspensive, the value of which last term I will soon explain.

I have based this proposition not alone upon pathological and clinical anatomy, but also upon the facts of experimentation. I have given, too, some contributions from pure anatomy which, to be sure, in certain respects, require confirmation, but such as they now are, they permit us to look into the mechanism by which the hemianæsthesia in question is produced.

There are some features relative to the totality of symptoms and their anatomical and physiological interpretation, that I have purposely left in shadow, so as not to overcrowd the picture. I propose now to recur to them.

I. First, let me in a few words recite the clinical characters of that kind of hemianæsthesia which I propose to call *cerebral hemianæsthesia*, in order to distinguish it from all other forms of obscuration or diminution of sensibility, the origin of which is not recognized as depending upon a lesion of the brain proper.

It is only lately that cerebral hemianæsthesia from gross organic lesion—"*coarse disease*," as H. Jackson, with a liberty quite English, terms it—has been the object of attentive study. The picture it presents is exactly that of hysterical hemianæsthesia; this last, being at present better known, will more naturally serve as a prototype.

Hysteria, you know, presents a *unilateral* anæsthesia. Total anæsthesia is relatively rare. An antero-posterior plane through the median line of the body marks the limit of insensibility, which line upon the trunk, however, is somewhat overstepped on the sternum in front, and on the spinal crest behind. This is a detail of secondary importance.

The head, the limbs, and the body on one side, then, are all affected at the same time. There may naturally be degrees in the functional disturbance, but more frequently it embraces all kinds of common sensibility; the sense of touch, of pain, and of temperature are often simultaneously obscured or suppressed.

The insensibility extends to the profound parts; it affects the muscles, which may be electrically excited without the patient's consciousness of it. The mucous membranes are not spared. Finally, let us add—and this is the point which above all others I just now desire to make prominent—hemianæsthesia does not include common sensation alone, it involves also the *sensorial apparatus* of the same side of the body affected with cutaneous anæsthesia, and that *sensorial hemianæsthesia* takes in, not only the nerves coming from the bulb, such as those of taste and hearing, but also the nerves of smell and vision, the origins of which are in the brain proper.

Such is the common picture of the hemianæsthesia of hysteria. If we compare the hemianæsthesia really cerebral with this, we will see a perfect resemblance, even to the smallest detail.

We have already carefully brought to light the resemblance as concerns common sensation,[1] and Magnan has done the same in that which concerns troubles of hearing, smell, and taste.[2] I see nothing to add to what has been said upon the subject. Lately we have been more particularly occupied with those phenomena which concern vision. In my service at Salpêtrière, Dr. Landolt has devoted himself to researches in that direction, the results of which merit brief mention.

It seems to me of interest to offer some facts showing that, even as relates to visual troubles (and this you will soon recognize as of great consequence), absolutely the same things occur in real cerebral lesions as with those simply hysterical. Abstraction seems to exhibit here its proverbial changeability; the unilateral amblyopia of hysterics differs in no essential character from the crossed cerebral amblyopia recognized as having an organic origin.

Let us first examine hysterical amblyopia.

II. 1st. Here diminution more or less pronounced, and sometimes (though rarely) absolute loss of vision upon the side corresponding to the hemianæsthesia, is the first easily recognized symptom.

2d. A more minute study develops the following peculiarities: There exist in the bottom of the eye no alterations appreciable by the opthalmoscope. The pupil and retina are entirely normal. Comparative examination of the posterior portions of the two eyes shows also no appreciable difference in their vascularization.

If the ophthalmoscope does not betray alterations in *amblyopia* of hysteria, it is not the same with subjective functional phenomena. This is what is learned through that method of examination.

---

[1] Charcot.—Lectures upon Maladies of the Nervous System, 1st ed., 1872.

[2] Magnan.—Upon Hemianæsthesia of General Sensibility and of the Special Senses in Chronic Alcoholism. Gaz. hebd., 1873, pp. 729 and 746.

3d. Visual acuteness, studied after ordinary rules, often shows itself reduced by one-half or even more.

4th. There exists a *general and concentric contraction of* the field of vision.

5th. Careful analysis has recognized certain peculiarities which deserve attention ; they concern the *concentric and general contraction of the field of vision for colors.*

Many authors, among others Galezowski, have heretofore remarked the frequent accompaniment of achromatopsia and dyschromatopsia with hysteria. These are the special points of observation made in my service by Landolt.

I would recall to you that in the normal state, all regions of the visual field are not, for some reason, equally apt in perception of colors. There are colors for which the visual field is physiologically more extended than for others, and these differences in the extent of the visual field always occur in the same subject according to the same law for each color. Thus the widest field of vision is for blue ; then yellow, then orange, red, green, and lastly violet, which is only perceived by the most central parts of the retina. Now, in the pathological condition with which we are occupied, the normal condition exists, though in various degrees exaggerated. Indeed the various circles which in this investigation correspond to the limits of vision for each color, are contracted concentrically in a more or less marked manner, but still based upon the law recognized for the normal state.

From this you can easily foresee the numerous combinations which may arise in cases of hysteria where this kind of amblyopia has attained a high degree. The violet circle may contract to nothing, then as the malady advances the same will occur consecutively with the green, red, and orange ; the yellow and blue remain to the last; observation demonstrates that these are the two colors for which sensitiveness is longest preserved in cases of hysteria. Finally, in extreme cases, it may happen that perception of all colors ceases, and then to the eyes of the patient colored objects would all become reduced to the appearance of a sepia drawing.

Such is the series of phenomena which we have over and

over observed in hysterical amblyopia. Now, these are all
met with in their different shades, in various cases of crossed
amblyopia accompanied with hemianæsthesia and arising
from a lesion in the centre of the brain, such as we have recently examined. The same is true of diminution of visual
acuteness ; of concentric and general contraction of the visual
field of colors, even where no pathognomonic lesions at the
bottom of the eye are appreciable with the ophthalmoscope,
etc.[1]

I insist especially upon this last characteristic, because it
permits a clear separation of the functional trouble from those
usually caused by intercranial, organic lesions. I allude to
the alterations at the bottom of the eye, easily discovered
with the ophthalmoscope, and commonly known under the
name of *papillary strangling* or *neuro-retinitis*, and which is
so frequently seen as a consequence of encephalic tumors,
whatever may be their nature or location,[2] and also following
various lesions acting more or less directly on the optic
bands.

In making known to you that crossed amblyopia is a consequence of lesions within the brain, I have stated a fact of
major importance for the theory of cerebral localization. But
it cannot escape you that this fact is in formal contradiction
to generally diffused ideas. Indeed, if the theory put forth in
1860, by Alb. de Graefe,[3] and which still appears to hold un-
divided sway, as witness an interesting work recently pub-

---

[1] New researches made for me by Landolt have demonstrated that contraction
of the field of vision for colors, in ovarian hysteria with hemianæsthesia, is always
experienced in both eyes at the same time ; only it is incomparably more pronounced in the eye corresponding to the side affected with the anæsthesia. The
same peculiarity is encountered in all cases, which have been examined in this respect, of *cerebral hemianæsthesia* arising from organic lesions. Therefore the
term *crossed amblyopia*, used in these lectures, will not be taken as absolutely
literal, since the obscuration of sight affects, unequally to be sure, both eyes.

[2] See upon this subject the interesting work of Dr. Annuske.—*Die Neuritis
Optica bei Tumor Cerebri*, in *Arch. für Ophthalmologie*, 19 Bd., Abth. III.,
1873, p. 165.

[3] A. de Graefe.—Gazette hebdomadaire, 1860, p. 708. See, also, Vorträge aus
der V. Graefe'schen Klinik. Monatsbl. f. Augenhlkde., 1865, Mai.

lished by Dr. Schoen,[1] be credited, it is not crossed amblyopia which determines exclusively unilateral lesions of the brain, but a different visual trouble, namely, *lateral homologous hemiopia ;* in other words, a cerebral lesion of the left substance of the brain should, according to the theory in question, produce suppression or obscuration of the right half of the visual field, and the reverse in case of a lesion in the right half of the brain.

I believe that I can protest against this theory as being at least too absolute, and I offer against it the following proposition : *cerebral lesions of the hemispheres which produce hemianæsthesia produce also crossed amblyopia, and not lateral hemiopia.*

I am not prepared, let it be well understood, to decide that lateral hemiopia is never the consequence of a lesion in the substance of the brain, but I am disposed to believe that such cases, if they really exist, are phenomena of contiguity—the effects, for example, of a more or less direct participation of the optic bands.   I do not believe that there now exists a single observation clearly showing, except in this way, the development of lateral hemiopia as a consequence of a lesion of the posterior part of the internal capsule or the foot of the diverging fibres, while a number of facts exist where such a lesion has produced *crossed amblyopia* with all the characteristics that we have just assigned to it.

III. We must give some details relative to the symptoms of *hemiopia* and the presumed anatomical cause of its development.

You know that this singular phenomenon, so often observed in clinic, has long since suggested an anatomical hypothesis according to which the optic nerves in man do not make a complete decussation in the optic chiasma, but that which is called a *semidecussation.*   That hypothesis is an old one.   It is generally attributed to Wollaston, but it is really due to *Newton*, who expressed it in 1704, in his *Treatise upon Optics*, and

---

[1] Schoen.—Archiv der Heilkunde, 1875, 1st Heft.

which Vater, in 1723, employed to explain three cases of hemiopia which had fallen under his observation.[1] I will recall the
hypothesis.

Among the nerve-tubes which form the bands of the optic
nerves there are those which, as has been said, decussate
in the chiasma and those which do not. (See Fig. 29.)
These last, that is, the non-decussating nerve-tubes, occupy
the external sides in the bands, in the chiasma, and also in the
optic nerves and the retina, whereas at all of these points the
fasciculi which decussate occupy the internal sides. It follows
that the non-decussating fasciculi, of the left band, for example,
being affected, would affect the left half of the retina of the
left eye, while the decussating fasciculi of the same band would
affect the left half of the right eye, the fasciculi of the right
optic bands operating of course after the same principle in-
versely.

In other words, the fasciculi which compose the optic band
of the left side would go to the left half of each retina, and
the reverse would occur with the nerve-fasciculi coming from
the optic bands of the right side.

It must be remembered that anatomically speaking this
arrangement of the optic nerve-fibres is entirely hypothetical.
If, indeed, various authors, among others Hannover,[2] Longet,
Cruveilhier, Henle,[3] and more recently Gudden,[4] have thought
themselves able to offer anatomical proof, there are others,
such as Biesiadecki,[5] E. Mandelstamm,[6] and Michel,[7] who contradict it, and appealing to the same order of arguments

[1] Knapp.—Archives of Scientific Medicine, New York, 1872.
[2] Hannover.—"Das Auge," Beiträge zur Anatomie, Physiologie, und Patholo-
gie dieses Organs, Leipzig, 1872.
[3] Henle.—Nervenlehre. Ueber die Kreutzung im Chiasma Nervorum Opticorum.
[4] Gudden.—Arch. für Ophthalmologie, 1874, t. 20, 2d Abth.
[5] E. Biesiadecki.—Ueber das Chiasma Nervorum Opticorum des Menschen und
der Thiere. Wiener Sitzber. d. math. Naturwiss. Classe B., d. 42 Jahrg. 1861,
p. 86.
[6] E. Mandelstamm.—"Ueber Sehnervenkreuzung und Hemiopie." Arch. für
Ophthalmologie, t. 16, 1873, p. 39.
[7] Michel.—Ueber den Bau des Chiasma Nervorum Opticorum. Same work, p.
59, Taf. I., Fig. IV. See also Bastian, The Lancet, 1874, July 25, p. 112.

attempt to demonstrate that the nerve-fibres of the optic nerves, even in man, submit to a complete decussation. In short, it may be said that at present the question is far from being settled. I repeat that the *semidecussation* is only an hypothesis; but that hypothesis explains, far better than any of its substitutes, all the facts observed in clinic. In the scheme herewith given it will be seen how easily it serves to interpret the various modes of hemiopia. (Fig. 29.)

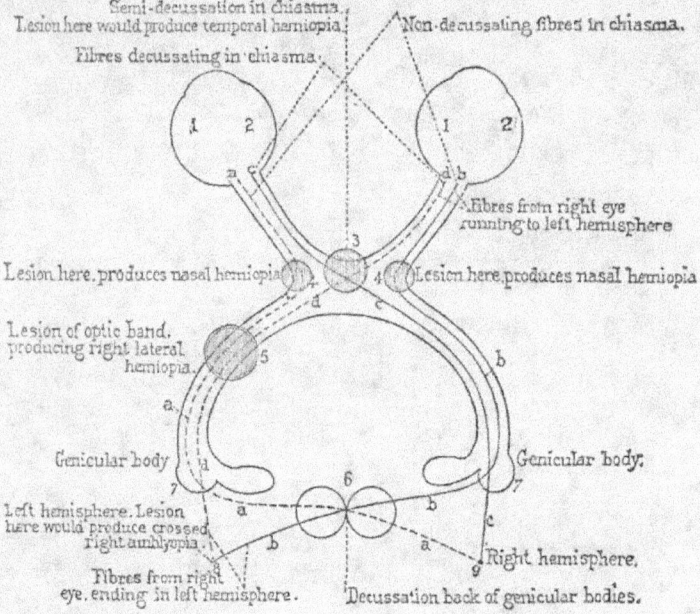

FIG. 29.—Scheme to explain the phenomena of lateral hemiopia and crossed amblyopia.

We will first consider *unilateral homologous hemiopia*, that which, according to writers, can occur only as the direct consequence of an intracerebral lesion of the brain. It is clear that according to the theory, a lesion situated at 5 in such way as to interrupt the tract of the fasciculi of the left optic band, those fibres which crossed in the chiasma (*d*), and also those which did not cross (*a*), would result in affecting the left half of each retina (*I I*), in other words, might obscure or completely suppress the entire extent of the visual field of the right side (*lateral right hemiopia*). *Lateral left hemiopia* would ensue from a lesion affecting in the same manner the optic band of the right side.

Thus speaks theory ; as for facts, there are numerous examples which demonstrate that lateral hemiopia is really the consequence of a lesion bearing upon one of the optic bands.[1] The effect will remain the same, no matter upon what part of the band, between its origin in the genicular body and its termination in the chiasma, the lesion occurs. Lateral hemiopia may also be produced not only by a lesion in the band itself, but also as a contiguous phenomenon in consequence of lesions—hemorrhage or tumors—developed in parts which are in more or less immediate relation with the tract, such, for example, as the lower part of the cerebral peduncle (*pes*) or in the pulvinar.

Other modes of hemiopia are not difficult to interpret. A lesion, a tumor, for example, situated at (3), that is, upon the median part of the chiasma in such way as to involve only the decussating optic fibres (*c, d*) might paralyze the left (1) half of the retina of the right eye as well as the right half (2) of the retina of the left eye, and so produce what is called temporal hemiopia. Saemisch foretold, in a case of this kind, while the patient still lived, that such was the location of the lesion, and autopsy fully justified his prediction.[2]

On the contrary, that hemiopia, called *nasal*, characterized by the suppression of the median portion of the field of vision, would be produced if the course of the direct fibres (*a, b*) only were interrupted, at the chiasma, for example, in consequence of lesions occupying each side symmetrically at the points (4, 4). This is a combination which is indeed rare. There exists, however, some examples ; among others one

---

[1] See, among others, the case of E. Müller in the Arch. für Ophthalmologie, VIII. Band 1, S. 160.

[2] See also E. Müller in Meissner's Jahresbericht, 1861, S. 458.

carefully described by Knapp.[1] In this case it resulted from a pressure upon the points indicated, by the anterior cerebral arteries and the posterior communicant artery enlarged and indurated by an atheromatous degeneration.

I will dwell no longer upon these forms of hemiopia, which do not at present directly interest us, but return to lateral hemiopia. It seems an established fact that this visual trouble is the necessary result of a lesion of the optic bands; it is also generally affirmed to be the necessary consequence of a lesion which may affect the optic nerve-fibres beyond the corpora geniculata (7) in their deep intracerebral tract (in 8, 9). In my opinion, clinical and pathological anatomy contradict that assertion—at all events, when made in too absolute a manner; and in this respect I can but repeat that which I just now have said; I do not believe that there now exists a solitary observation showing, beyond doubt, the development of lateral hemiopia in consequence of an intracerebral lesion *outside of all participation of the optic tracts*, whereas facts exist where a lesion of the posterior part of the internal capsule, or the foot of the diverging fibres, has produced hemianæsthesia, and at the same time crossed amblyopia, a visual trouble very diverse from hemiopia.

That being the case, how can we understand, in a schematic view, that effect of a cerebral lesion, while at the same time we recognize the incontestable fact of hemiopia being the consequence of a lesion of the optic bands?

To this end a slight modification of the common scheme will suffice. It is generally admitted that the nerve-fibres coming from the right eye and the left eye which compose each of the optic bands continue their course beyond the corpora geniculata uninterruptedly into the very depths of the corresponding hemispheres, and that view accords with the prevailing idea that a lesion of the optic nerve-fibres in their intracerebral course is equivalent to a lesion of the optic bands, and consequently produces hemiopia.

I propose to admit, on the contrary, that only the fasciculi

---

[1] Arch. of Scientific and Practical Medicine, 1873, p. 293.

of the bands which decussate in the chiasma (*c*, *d*) reach their
profound depths, whatever they may be, without new decussation ; whereas the direct fasciculi do completely decussate
beyond the corpora geniculata, before entering into the
depth of the hemispheres (8, 9) ; this occurs upon an undeter-
mined point of the median line, perhaps in the tubercula
quadrigemina.   From that arrangement it would result that
the fasciculi (*b*, d), reunited, for example, in a point of the
left hemisphere (8), would represent the totality of the fibres
coming from the retina of the right eye, and that the fasciculi
(*a*, *c*) would represent the totality of fibres coming from the
left eye.   The optic fibres, according to that, in their profound course, are at length all reduced to the type of complete decussating fibres, and one can comprehend that, in an
apparatus so constructed, a lesion of the optic bands would
produce lateral hemiopia, although a lesion situated deeply
in the substance of the brain would to the contrary produce
crossed amblyopia.

I give you this hypothesis for whatever it is worth.   At
present it has no anatomical base.   But at all events it furnishes, if I am not deceived, an easy means of very simply
representing the tolerably complex facts revealed by clinical
observation.

ELEVENTH LECTURE.

ORIGIN OF THE CEREBRAL PORTION OF THE OPTIC NERVES.

Summary:—Relations of Crossed Amblyopia and Sensitive Hemianæsthesia, Resulting from a Lesion of the Internal Capsule.—
Cerebral Origin of the Optic Nerves.—Diverging Fibres of Reil.—
Radiating Cortico-optic Fasciculi.—Anterior Fibres (Anterior Roots
of the Thalami Optici); Middle Fibres (Lateral Expansion); Posterior Fibres (Cerebral Expansion of the Optic Nerves); Anatomical
Relations between the Cerebral Expansion of the Optic Nerves and
the Centripetal Portions of the Radiating Fibres (Sensitive Hemianæsthesia).—Optic Bands.—Origin of the External Root (Thalami
Optici); External Geniculate Bodies, Anterior Tubercula Quadrigemina.—Origins of the Internal Root (Internal Geniculate Bodies,
Posterior Tubercula Quadrigemina).—Relation between the Mass
of Gray Substance and the Gray Cortex of the Encephalon.—Cortico-
optic Radiating Fasciculi.—Effects of Lesions of the Anterior Tubercula Quadrigemina.—Facts of Lateral Hemiopia of Supposed
Intra-cerebral Origin.

GENTLEMEN:

I hope that I have demonstrated the existence of crossed amblyopia as a symptom of lesion in the posterior part of the internal capsule, or of the corresponding irradiations of the foot of the diverging fibres.

At the same time I have attempted to prove de Graefe's proposition, that homologous hemiopia might be (crossed amblyopia excluded) the only functional trouble of vision following a lesion of the cerebral hemispheres, to be at least too sweeping, and that the arguments upon which it rests ought to be completely revised.

I now wish to examine whether normal anatomy can explain why the sensorial trouble in question, that is, crossed amblyopia, is a frequent, as it were habitual, accompaniment of sensitive hemianæsthesia resulting from a lesion of the internal capsule.

This hemianæsthesia of common sensibility, you remember, may be produced through the existence of a fasciculus of *direct* centripetal fibres, that is, fibres not stopping in the gray ganglia of the central masses, and which, upon issuing from the internal capsule, form the very posterior portion of the diverging fibres.

Does there exist a connection, a more or less immediate relation, between that sensitive fasciculus and the sensorial fasciculi designed to put the apparatus of vision in communication with the gray cortex of the brain? To enter upon this question it is first necessary to study the origin of the profound or cerebral part of the optic nerves. We will examine this difficult subject, which is still obscure in more than one point. I must not, however, omit giving you the principal outlines, if only to indicate the direction in which our future researches should be made, and where pathological anatomy will very likely be called to play a dominant part.

According to the general plan, the encephalic nerves ought to encounter, before penetrating the brain itself, one or more masses of gray substance, which it is agreed to call the *ganglions of origin*, and the expansions arising from these ganglia put these nerves in an indirect *rapport* with the gray cortex of the cerebral hemispheres.

A priori, there is nothing to induce belief that the optic nerves escape the rule. In fact, they do not escape it, but their distributions are very complicated and ill-known, especially in some of the details.

I. I will pause an instant to note the construction of a portion of the diverging fibres of Reil.[1]

---

[1] The various fasciculi, peduncular or otherwise, which form the diverging fibres, (*fibres convergentes* of Luys) (*système de projection de 1ᵉ ordre* of Meynert) compose the greater portion of the white central mass called centrum ovale, which the gray cortex of the hemispheres envelops and encloses like a purse. They, however, do not represent the totality of that mass. It contains, beyond these, fasciculi entirely foreign to the preceding, but which mix with them. These last fasciculi constitute that which Meynert calls the *system of association*. One may distinguish in a general way the two orders of fasciculi which compose this system.

In the scheme which I present to you and which is borrowed from Huguenin (loc. cit., pl. 69, page 93), the ablation

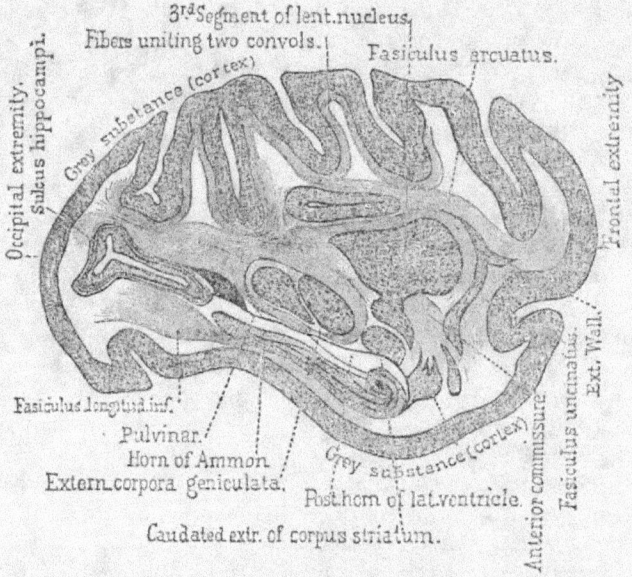

FIG. 30 —Antero-posterior section of a monkey's brain (*Cercocebus cinomolgus*) showing the connecting fibres of the brain.—(*Meynert*, Stricker's Hand-book.)

of the superior parts of the hemispheres, including the corpus callosum, has laid bare the ventricular cavities. You will

---

One kind consists of commissures which unite the homologous parts of the two hemispheres. Such, for example, are the corpora callosa and the anterior commissure. The others are composed of fibres having a general antero-posterior direction, which bring into relation the various points of the same hemisphere. Fig. 30, borrowed from Meynert (loc. cit., Fig. 233), representing the anterior section of the brain of a monkey (*Cercocebus cinomolgus*), very well exhibits the direction of the principal fasciculi of the antero-posterior system of association. There are to be seen the fibres uniting two convolutions (*fibræ propriæ*), well described by Gratiolet, the *fasciculus arcuatus*, the fibres of which extend beneath the corpus callosum from the occipital to the frontal lobe ; the inferior longitudinal fasciculus which joins the occipital lobe to the extremity of the sphenoidal lobe, and finally, the *fasciculus uncinatus*, which runs nearly vertical and which joins the frontal to the sphenoidal lobe.

notice particularly the inferior part, or the posterior cornu of
the ventricle which here plays an important rôle in topography (Fig. 32).

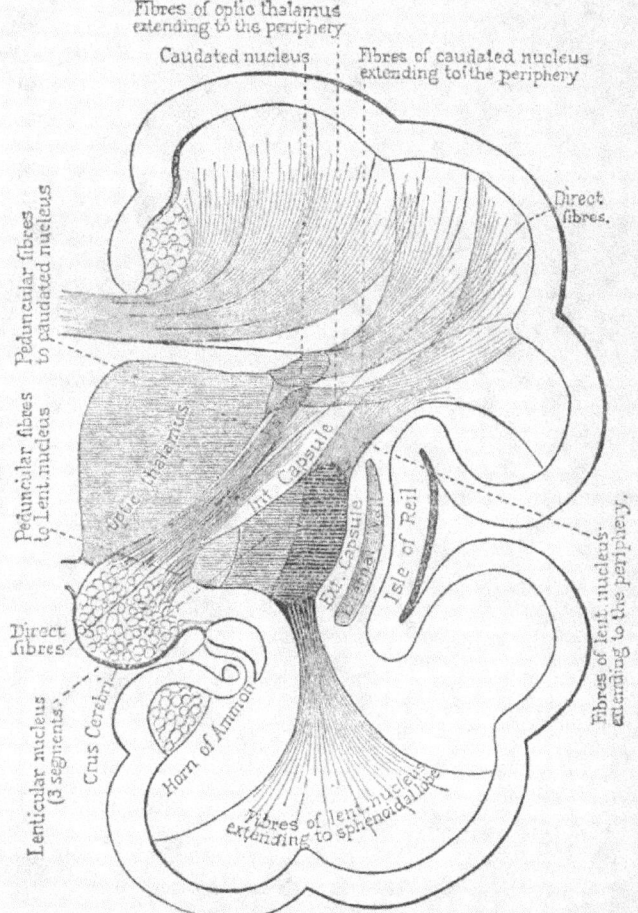

FIG. 31.—Scheme illustrative of the different orders of peduncular fibres.—(*Huguenin.*)

The caudated ganglion has been detached and its outlines
are represented by a dotted line; its diverging fibres, that is

to say, the plane of the cortico-striated radiating fibres, have also been removed.   Thus is uncovered the plane of the cortico-optic radiating fibres. In these last fasciculi it is possible to distinguish three groups of fibres : 1st, the anterior ones called anterior roots of the thalami-optici (Vordere Stiel), they are directed towards the frontal regions ; 2d, others are middle or lateral ; 3d, and finally, the posterior ones are designated by Gratiolet, who first[1] well studied them, under the name of optic cerebral expansions, or expansion of the optic nerves (*Sehstrahlungen*).   The fasciculi of the last group, which are the special object of our study, are separated from the cavity of the posterior cornu only by the ependymus and the *tapetum*, a special expansion of the splenium of the corpus callosum.

It is in this same region, but on a deeper plane, that the cerebral expansions of the fasciculi of centripetal fibres are spread, the lesion of which produces sensitive hemianæsthesia of cerebral origin.   There exists, then, a relation of propinquity, of contiguity, between these fasciculi and the optic expansions, and that relation would well explain anatomically the frequent coexistence of hemianæsthesia and crossed amblyopia if it could be well established that those fasciculi which bear the name of optic expansions are really a more or less direct prolongation of the optic nerves.

II. We will make a little digression upon this point in order to ascertain what is known about the gray ganglia at the base of the encephalon, outside of the brain proper, where the optic nerves originate.

Here it seems proper to examine the exterior architecture of the parts which we are about to consider.

After detaching the entire isthmus from the encephalon, leaving attached the thalami optici, an examination of the posterior face of the preparation thus obtained will discover as follows : 1st, anteriorly, on each side, are the thalami optici, which separate the third ventricles ; 2d, posteriorly, the

---

[1] See Gratiolet, Anat. comparée, t. II., p. 181 et suiv. Luys, loc. cit., p. 173.

tubercula quadrigemina, both anterior and posterior ; 3d, externally, the anterior conjunctive fibres connecting by their internal extremities with the anterior tubercula quadrigemina,

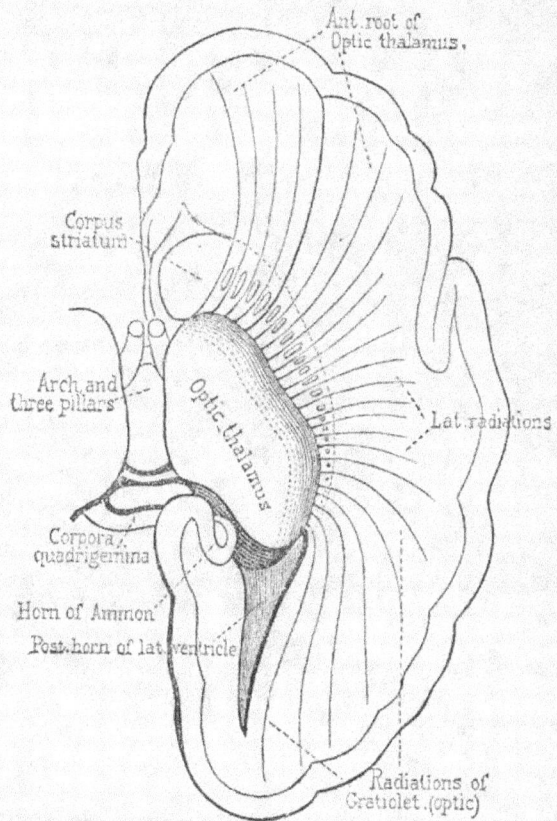

FIG. 32.—Radiations from the thalamus opticus.—(*Huguenin.*)

the posterior conjunctive fibres connecting with the posterior tubercula quadrigemina. Then, in the same region, by raising the posterior extremity of the thalami optici, or *pulvinar*, may be seen, internally, the internal geniculate body, and externally, a gray mass, somewhat more voluminous, which is the external geniculate body.

Behind and above these parts are to be seen the loop of Reil, the *processus cerebelli ad testes*, the cerebral peduncles, the restiform bodies, and the middle cerebral peduncles.

The internal and external geniculate bodies are notably the first two ganglia of gray substance with which the optic nerves enter into *rapport* on their way to the encephalon. The optic nerves posterior to the chiasma take the name of *optic tracts*, or *optic bands*, and in the posterior two-thirds they are divided into two tracts which may be considered as roots, the one internal, the other external.

The *external* is most voluminous and also most important. It furnishes several fibres which run to various gray ganglia. 1st. There can be seen a fasciculus which goes to the external geniculate body. These bodies are a tolerably voluminous mass of gray substance, enclosing ganglionic cells, stellate or fusiform, of considerable dimensions, and which are to be found well represented in the work of Henle (Fig. 177, p. 249). 2d. A second fasciculus, situated within the preceding, enters the inferior portion of the *thalamus* about twelve millimètres anterior to the extremity of the *pulvinar*. Upon a transverse section, such as is represented in the work of Meynert (Fig. 249, II. R.), the fasciculus in question is situated between the external geniculate body and the foot of the peduncle. The existence of this fasciculus, affirmed by Gratiolet, is also very explicitly recognized by Meynert, Henle, and Huguenin. 3d. A third fasciculus which, according to Gratiolet, should be the most apparent and best known of the roots of the optic nerves, winds around the external geniculate bodies and enters the anterior tuberculum quadrigeminus of the corresponding side.[1] The description which Gratiolet has given of this, confirmed also by Vulpian and Huguenin,[2] is perfectly exact as concerns the most of mam-

---

[1] Gratiolet, loc. cit., p. 180.
[2] Huguenin, Westphall's Arch., V. Bd., 1st Heft, 2d Heft, 1875.

mifera.[1] It does not hold true in the same degree for the monkey; and in man, though the fasciculus exists, it can be anatomically demonstrated only by great care.[2]

It is thus seen that the *external roots* of the optic nerves take their origin in three ganglia of gray substance, to wit: 1st, the thalami optici; 2d, the external geniculate bodies; 3d, the anterior tubercula quadrigemina (nates). Such certainly are the principal sources of the optic nerves in man, and with a great number of animals they are probably the only ones; at least this seems to be established by the interesting experiments of Gudden,[3] consisting of the extirpation of the eyeballs of very young rabbits. In the animals thus operated upon, when killed some months thereafter, it was observed that consecutive atrophy had ensued in the central parts upon the anterior tubercula quadrigemina (nates), the thalami optici, and the external geniculate bodies; on the other hand, the posterior tubercula quadrigemina (testes) and the internal geniculate bodies did not participate in the atrophy.

The *internal roots*, though less important than the external, should not be neglected, especially when relating to man. You know that they are connected with the internal geniculate bodies. These internal geniculate bodies contain only rudimentary nerve-cells (Henle), and consequently cannot be considered as a centre in the same sense as can the external geniculate bodies. The nerve-fasciculi of the internal root, it may be either after traversing the geniculate bodies, or by a direct course, proceed to a final termination at the anterior tubercula quadrigemina (nates).

Quite recently Huguenin (*Arch. für Psychiatric*, 1875, V. Bd., Fasc. 2, p. 344) has maintained that the internal roots of

---

[1] For brains of the rabbit and dog, see plate, Gudden's work (Arch. of Ophthal., XX., 1875); for brain of cat, the plates of Forel (*Beiträge zur Kenntniss der Thalamus Opticus*). Sitzbericht. der k. Akad., LXVI. Bd., 1872, T. II., Fig. 10.

[2] A fourth fasciculus, situated outside of the one which stops in the external geniculate body, is spread upon the thalamus and takes part in forming the *Stratum zonale*. Previously indicated by Arnold and Gratiolet, this fasciculus is described and represented also by Meynert, p. 436.

[3] Gudden.—Arch. für Ophthalmol., XX.

the optic nerves, in man at least, are in anatomical *rapport* with the posterior tubercula quadrigemina, either directly or by the intermediation of the internal geniculate bodies. According to that, the posterior tubercula quadrigemina could not, in man, be excluded, as it seems to be in animals, from the apparatus of the optic nerves. This is not in contradiction with the teaching of certain facts concerning gray tabetic induration of the optic nerves. Quite recently, in an ataxied woman—blind for fifteen years—gray induration of the optic nerves could be followed beyond the chiasma along the optic bands quite to the geniculate bodies. The tubercula quadrigemina, the anterior (nates), as well as the posterior (testes), had very nearly retained the white color of the normal state, but they both were manifestly reduced in size (case of Magdaliat[1]). I have observed several cases, all similar to the preceding.

We must now examine how the various masses of gray substance which have been enumerated are brought into relation with the gray cortex of the encephalon. The connection is established, as I have shown, by a system of fibres which constitute the most posterior portion of the radiations of the thalami optici (cortico-optic diverging fasciculi), and which are sometimes called the *optic radiations of Gratiolet*. You can follow these somewhat complex anatomical details in the following plate, which I borrow from the work of Meynert, and which represents the brain of a monkey (*Cercocebus cinomolgus*) (Fig. 33).

It can there be seen how the fasciculi of fibres, or radiations, leaving the external geniculate bodies, the internal geniculate bodies, the pulvinar, and the anterior tubercula quadrigemina (these last by the intermediation of the anterior conjunctive arms), go by a recurrent way to associate with a medullary fasciculus which is only a collection of the *direct peduncular* centripetal fibres that we have already described (Lectures VIII. and IX., Fig. 26), and upon which the common sensibility of the opposite side of the body depends.

---

[1] The anterior and posterior conjunctive arms were remarkably atrophied; they had a heavy white color, a little tinted with yellow.

With that collection of fibres are doubtless mingled other fibres coming from the olfactive tract by way of the anterior commissure, the extremities of which, according to the descriptions of Burdach and Gratiolet, are directed posteriorly

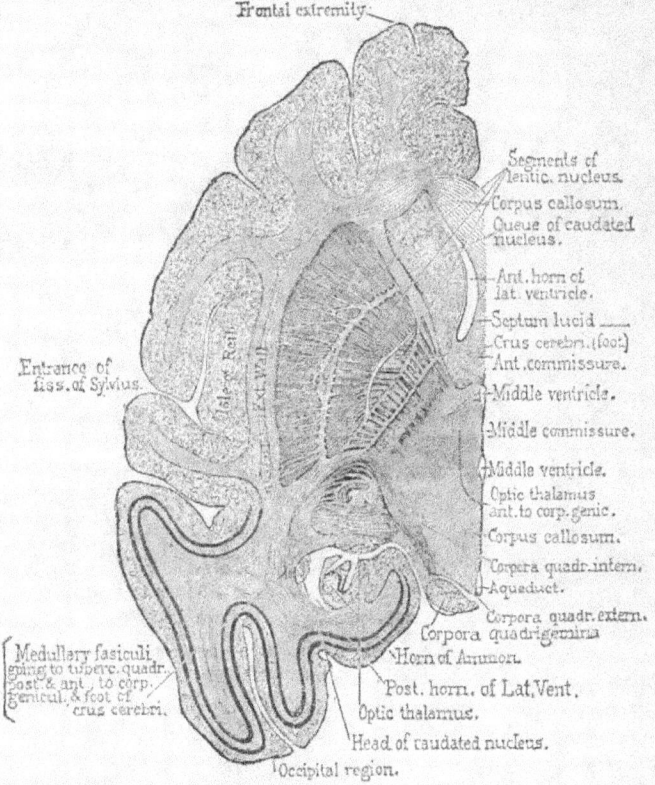

FIG. 33.—Antero-posterior horizontal section of the left hemisphere of a monkey's brain (*Cercocebus cinomolgus*).—(*Meynert*, Stricker's Handbook.)

into the substance of the occipital and sphenoidal lobes. Clinical facts lead to the belief that there also are mingled decussating nerve-fibres connected with the auditory and gustatory nerves. If that arrangement, now altogether hypothetical, should come to be anatomically verified, it can be understood how crossed obscuration of the smell, taste, and hearing should, in the same manner as amblyopia, be an ordinary symptom of *cerebral hemianæsthesia*.[1]

The encephalic region to which I have drawn your attention, and which responds to the most posterior part of the foot of the radiating fibres (*couronne rayonnante*), may be considered, then, as a highway where, in the depths of the encephalon, are encountered, within a very narrow space, all the sensitive and sensorial lines of travel. This is a highway ; it is not a centre. The cerebral centre, properly speaking, should be sought in the prolongations of the medullary fibres, in the gray cortex of the occipital and sphenoidal lobes.

We shall return to this point in connection with localizations in the cortical system.

III. You might have observed in the preceding anatomical *exposé* that the tubercula quadrigemina seem to furnish the only point where the fasciculi of the optic nerves, after their decussation in the chiasma, again approach each other upon the median line. This is the point where that supplementary decussation is effected, which, according to my hypothesis, would reduce the optic nerve to the same footing as other nerves. That is a question which at present seems difficult to resolve by exclusively anatomical means. Upon the median line, between the tubercula quadrigemina, numerous decussations of fibres are without doubt anatomically demonstrated. But it cannot be decided whether these decussated fibres are really in connection with the optic nerves, and especially whether they are the prolongations of optic fibres non-decussating in the chiasma. Experimentation, and above all pathological anatomy, should certainly have the first place in the solution of this question. The experiments of Flourens have already shown that with mammifera and with birds, the ablation of the optic tubercles produce amblyopia or crossed amaurosis. But this is with animals in which the

---

[1] According to the theory, cerebral hemianæsthesias should be distinguished from those dependent upon a lesion of the protuberance or the cerebral peduncles (crus cerebri) by non-participation in the last case of vision or smell.

ocular axes are directed externally and in which the decussation in the chiasma is doubtless complete.

With man the elements for the solution of the problem are as yet defective. With him lesions of the tubercula quadrigemina are not rare, but they ordinarily are bilateral, and consequently producing bilateral blindness, they can prove nothing. In fact, it is still a question whether lesions of the anterior tubercula quadrigemina will, like a lesion of the optic bands, produce lateral hemiopia, or if, on the contrary, they will produce crossed amblyopia, as would be in keeping with my hypothesis. In favor of my hypothesis, I can as yet cite but one case, reported by Dr. Bastian, and in which a unilateral lesion of the anterior tubercula quadrigemina had produced crossed amblyopia.

But that fact is at present the only one, and besides it is related with too little detail to be received as decisive.[1]

IV. It remains to ascertain if crossed amblyopia is the only kind of functional trouble of the vision which can be produced by a lesion of the brain proper, or if, on the contrary, hemiopia may not also follow as a consequence of certain pathological localizations in the hemisphere. That is a point which, I think, no one is at present competent to decide. I incline, however, in the absence of contradictory autopsies, to believe that in most instances of hemiopia which have been ascribed to a lesion of the brain, the lesion has either not occupied the deep regions of the hemisphere, or that it has extended to the basilar portions in such manner as to involve more or less directly one or the other of the optic bands.

To show that deep lesions of the brain produce hemiopia—lateral hemiopia—cases are specially cited where the visual disturbance is suddenly developed upon an apoplectic stroke, and where, at the same time, the limbs of one side are affected with motor hemiplegia, and sometimes also with anæsthesia. Nothing is better established in clinic than facts of this kind,

---

[1] H. C. Bastian, The Lancet, 1874, 25th July.

CEREBRAL PORTION OF THE OPTIC NERVES.   113

of which Schoen, quite recently, in an interesting work, has cited several examples.[1]   But the conduction of the autopsies have to the present been faulty, and it may be queried if the lesion found in these cases occupied really the deep brain, or, on the contrary, the base of the encephalon.   It seems established, you have not forgotten, that destruction or compression of one of the optic bands produces lateral hemiopia ; and, on the other hand, the anatomical relation which exists between the bands and certain parts of the isthmus, such, among others, as the crura cerebri, is well known. Such being the case, it could not be otherwise than that a lesion properly localized, as, for example, in a crus cerebri, might result in producing at the same time lateral hemiopia and motor hemiplegia, and perhaps also hemianæsthesia.   Hemorrhage, suddenly developed in the substance of the posterior part of the thalami optici, might, as can be understood, be followed with the same effect.   It is evident that these diverse combinations are only phenomena of propinquity.

In any case, it should be known that among instances which have been reported of lateral hemiopia of supposed intracerebral origin, there are a certain number which in some respects do not conform to the interpretations that I have proposed.   Such, among others, are those where right lateral hemiopia develops itself in concert with aphasia, and sometimes also with various modifications of the sensibility or motion of the limbs of the right side of the body.[2]

These facts do not constitute a homogeneous group ; the first category includes a form peculiar to *migraine*,[3] that is, symptoms essentially transitory, returning by accesses, and above all marked by scintillations, vertigo, more or less marked lateral hemiopia, and sometimes also with a certain

---

[1] Arch. der Heilkunde, p. 19, 1875.

[2] Various cases of this kind have recently been related by Bernhardt (Berliner klin. Wochen., 32, 1872, and Centralblatt, 1872, 39), and by Schoen (loc. cit.). See also H. Jackson, A Case of Hemiopia with Hemianæsthesia and Hemiplegia, in the Lancet, Aug. 29, 1874, p. 306.

[3] See respecting this form of migraine the works of Tissot, Labarraque, Piorry, and Latham (on *Nervous Sick Headache*, Cambridge, 1873), and above all the recent work of Ed. Liveing (on *Megrim*, etc., London, 1873).

degree of aphasia and numbness in the face and limbs of the right side. Headache, nausea, and vomiting usually end the attack. It is clear that these cases cannot be ascribed to a durable, material alteration. It is not thus with the cases of the second category, where the concurrence of aphasia, hemiplegia, and hemiopia remain permanent.[1]

At present I do not see how these various cases, revealed by clinic, can be anatomically explained upon the hypothesis of a single lesion. I can only call attention to the difficulties, the solution of which is reserved to the future.

---

[1] It can be understood that a voluminous tumor might produce all the results noted in both categories, and it has happened in a case recently published by Hirschberg in the Archives of Virchow (Virchow's Arch., T. 65, 1 Heft, p. 116). This patient had, besides very characteristic right lateral hemiopia, aphasia, and hemiplegia of the right limbs. Upon autopsy there was found in the substance of the left frontal lobe, a tumor the size of an apple, of the kind called vascular glioma. The optic tract of the *left side was very flattened*. The views entertained in the present chapter find a confirmation in that fact, since the hemiopia there noted may belong to compression of the optic tract.

TWELFTH LECTURE.

SECONDARY DEGENERATION.

Summary:—Anterior or Lenticulo-Striated Region of the Central Masses (Anterior Two-thirds of Internal Capsule, the Caudated and Lenticular Ganglia).—Influence of Lesions in these Regions upon the Production of Motor Hemiplegia.—Experimental Facts.—Accord between these and the Facts of Human Pathology.—Difference between the Lesions of the Caudated Ganglion and those of the Anterior Part of the Internal Capsule.—Secondary Degenerations, or Descending Scleroses.—Lesions which Produce them; Importance of the Locality and Extent of these Lesions.—Characteristics of Descending Scleroses; Extent; Appearance of the Lesion upon the Crus Cerebri, the Protuberance, the Anterior Pyramid, and the Lateral Fasciculus of the Spinal Cord.—Analogies and Differences between Lateral Sclerosis from Cerebral Cause, and Primitive Fasciculated Sclerosis of the Lateral Fasciculi.—Symptoms Belonging to Secondary Sclerosis; Motor Impotency, Permanent Contractions.—Muscular Atrophy Produced by Extension of the Lateral Sclerosis to the Cornua of the Gray Substance.—Descending Sclerosis Following a Lesion of the Cortex.—Demonstration of the Direct Peduncular Fibres; Anatomico-Pathological Facts.—The Locations of Cortical Lesions which Produce Secondary Degenerations Correspond to the Locations of Centres called Psycho-Motor.

GENTLEMEN:

We must again turn to the *anterior regions of the central masses*, for the purpose of studying more carefully the anatomical and pathologico-physiological effects of lesions occurring in that locality.

That region, which may be called the *lenticulo-striated*, in contradistinction to the posterior or *lenticulo-optic* region, embraces, you remember, 1st, the anterior two-thirds of the white tract called the internal capsule ; 2d, internally from this, the large extremity or head of the caudated ganglion ; 3d, outside, by the side of the island of Reil, the anterior two-thirds nearly of the lenticulate ganglion.

Observation, and that many times repeated, demonstrates as I have already remarked in the course of these lectures Lectures VIII. and IX., pp. 70 and 71), that common motor hemiplegia, unaccompanied by derangement of sensibility, is the almost inevitable consequence of even the smallest lesions occurring in the various parts which I have enumerated, provided always that the lesions in question produce the de-

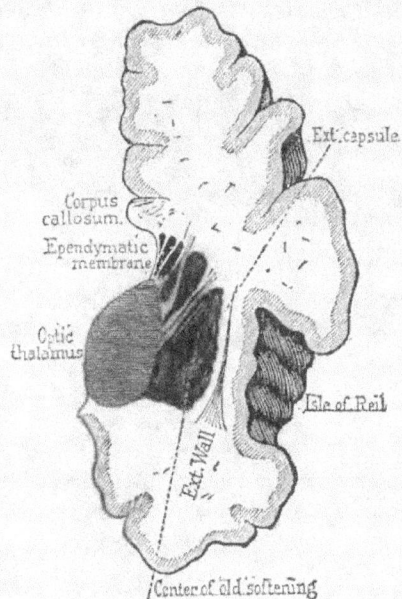

FIG. 34.—An old softening of the middle portion of the caudated ganglion and the internal capsule. (*Right side.*)

struction or the sudden compression of the nerve-elements of the affected area, instead of merely a slowly effected displacement, as is often seen in the case of tumors.

I called attention to an important distinction which should be established. This is, that lesions, even extensive and deep, which remain limited to the gray ganglia (caudated and lenticular ganglia), produce, as a general rule, symptoms relatively slight and transient, while lesions comparatively slight, which involve the white tract (internal capsule), give rise to a motor hemiplegia, not only very decided, but also of long duration and often incurable (Fig. 34).

Let us try and ascertain the reason of these differences. First, concerning the intensity of the paralytic symptoms in cases of lesions of the internal capsule compared to that mild degree in cases of lesions limited to the gray ganglia ; then we will examine the transitory character of hemiplegia in the last kind of cases as contrasted with the permanence of the same symptom which almost invariably results from lesions of the internal capsule.

I. Concerning the first point, I will remind you again of the anatomical construction of the internal capsule. That tract embraces : 1st. The *direct peduncular fibres*—that is, those originating beneath the gray cortex, and which enter the inferior portion of the crura cerebri without having entered into relation with the lenticular or caudated gray ganglia. 2d. The *indirect peduncular fibres*, which, on the contrary, originate in the lenticular or caudated ganglia, and have no connection with the gray cortex. For the moment we will leave unnoticed those fasciculi of fibres which extend from the cortical substance to the gray ganglia of the central mass.

We will suppose that the various peduncular fibres, direct and indirect, are centrifugal, and that they transmit to the periphery the motor influence developed, it may be, in the gray cortex of the brain, or in the lenticular and caudated gray ganglia.

With this hypothesis it is easy to comprehend that a small lesion of the internal capsule, especially near its inferior part, in the vicinity of the foot of the cerebral peduncle, where all the fibres are reassembled in a narrow space, would, at one blow, suppress the influence of the gray cortex and that of the two gray ganglia ; while, on the contrary, a lesion limited to the lenticular ganglion would leave free the action of the caudated ganglion and that of the gray cortex. The effects of various combinations of this sort which might happen can easily be imagined ; lesion of the caudated ganglion, of certain regions of the gray cortex, of the two gray ganglia, with or without the participation of the peduncular fibres of the internal capsule, etc.

I attach no more importance to this theoretical view than is permissible. It adapts itself well to the facts obtained by clinical observation upon man, and I will add also that it is in no part contradicted (you may judge for yourselves) by experiments made with animals.

For a long time it has been known [1] that with the majority of animals motor disturbances produced by the methodic destruction of various parts of the encephalon, particularly of the brain, differ considerably in a general way from similar pathological lesions of corresponding parts in man.

In the interpretation of these experimental facts, and in their application to human pathology, there should be taken into account, among other things, the greater or less inferiority of the species of animals and the more or less advanced age. Thus, the entire ablation of a cerebral hemisphere of a pigeon (and still more marked, of course, with a reptile) would produce no trouble which could be compared to hemiplegia. It is nearly the same with the rabbit. A feebleness slightly noticeable in the limbs of one side of the body is the only consequence of such a lesion in the rabbit. Standing and jumping are still possible, even though the entire brain has been destroyed, provided always that the protuberance remains intact.[2] With the dog, the results become notably different. From the last experiments made in the laboratory of Vulpian, by Carville and Duret, the results of methodic ablation of the various parts of the dog's brain greatly resemble those observed in cases of corresponding lesions of the cerebral hemisphere in man.

If the experiments were made upon the monkey, it is probable that the resemblance would be still more manifest and complete.

Here is a brief *exposé* of the principal results obtained by

---

[1] See upon this subject Longet.—Traité de physiologie, t. III., p. 431, and Vulpian.—Leçons sur la physiologie générale, etc., p. 676.

[2] Vulpian, Longet.

the experiments of Carville and Duret : 1st. In the dog, ablation of the gray substance of the central cortex of those regions called *motor centres* produced a temporary weakness (*paresis*) of the limbs upon the opposite side. 2d. The extirpation of the caudated ganglion produced an analogous but more marked paresis. Nothing can at present be said of the lenticular ganglion, the ablation of which, owing to its topographical position, could not be effected ;[1] 3d. If, on the contrary, the lesion be made upon the inferior part of the internal capsule, it produces in both fore and hind limbs of the opposite side, not only a simple paresis, but a well-marked motor paraly-

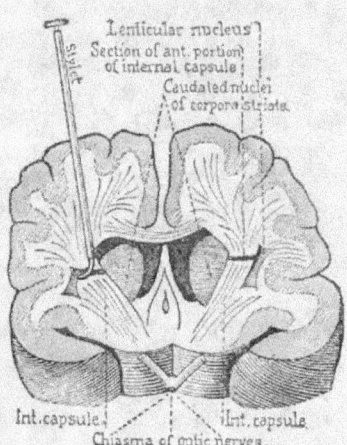

FIG. 35.—Transverse section of a dog's brain, five millimètres anterior to the optic chiasma. (*Operation of Veyssière.*)

sis which resembles the hemiplegia in man resulting from lesions of the same parts (Fig. 35). Held suspended by the skin of the back, the animal thus operated on could still stand on the sound limbs, but the affected ones hung flaccid, inert, and no longer capable of any movement except that which was purely reflex.

In short, you see from these interesting researches, which are worthy of multiplication, that the contradiction long since noticed between animals and man, relative to the influence of various parts of the hemisphere of the brain upon movement of the opposite limbs—that contradiction, I say, seems no longer to exist when the specimen for the comparison is relatively high in the animal scale. (Fig. 36.)

Perhaps it is not here out of the way to recall that even in

[1] In this respect it is difficult to utilize the experiments of Nothnagel with caustic injections. These injections must almost necessarily produce phenomena of excitation, which assuredly introduce a complication.

the dog—the result of experiments by both Carville and
Duret and Veyssière—lesions of the posterior part of the internal capsule produced crossed hemianæsthesia the same as
with man.

II. I think the previous considerations may render plain
the reason why hemiplegias resulting from destructive lesions

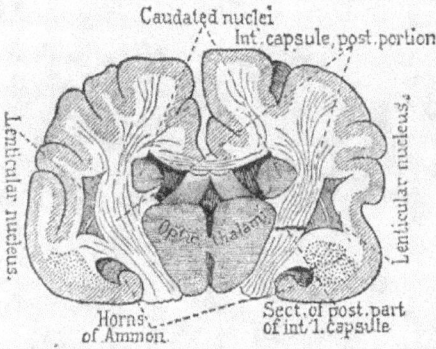

FIG. 36.—Transverse section of a dog's brain on a plane with the tubercula mammillaria.—(*Carville and Duret*.)

confined to the substance of the gray ganglia are as a rule
temporary, while those resulting from lesions in the substance
of the internal capsule are, on the contrary, of longer duration, and often even absolutely incurable.

Through the hypothesis proposed, it can easily be understood how the lenticular and caudated ganglia and the regions
called the motor centres in the gray cortex of the hemispheres
could mutually supplement each other in their functions, so
long as the conducting fasciculi which form the capsule have
preserved their integrity, and could continue to maintain the
relations of any one of the gray centres in question with the
peripheric parts ; whereas this could not take place if the
continuity of these fasciculi had been decidedly interrupted.

I will add that in all probability this supplementing may be
established not only between the various gray ganglia, but
also between the various parts of the same ganglion.   It is

demonstrated, at least as concerns the caudated ganglion of the corpus striatum, that partially destructive lesions affecting the most diverse regions of the ganglion are uniformly expressed by a more or less marked and transitory, but total hemiplegia; that is, affecting at the same time both the face and the limbs. In this respect there can be distinguished no difference between the head, the tail, or the middle part of the caudated ganglion. It would thus seem that H. Jackson was correct in remarking that each parcel of the striated body represented in miniature the entire body. Moreover, experimentation gives results in conformity with those furnished by clinical observation, in showing that partial excitation of the caudated ganglion, however effected, always produces movements of the entire opposite side of the body, and never disassociated movements; localized, for example, in one limb, or in a portion of a limb.[1]

In case of a destructive lesion of the internal capsule, a slow regeneration of the nerve-elements may, on the contrary, permit the gradual re-establishment of the functions. Now, that labor of restitution, if it is really sometimes accomplished, most certainly is not always so; it occurs only as an exception. It is placed beyond doubt, indeed, by very numerous observations, that those lesions which to a certain extent destroy the motor fibres of the internal capsule, have, as an almost necessary consequence, the production of a *fascicular lesion* which, commencing immediately below the site of the lesion, can be traced in the corresponding side to the foot of the peduncle, along the protuberance, and the anterior pyramid to the level of the bulbular decussation, and beneath this into the spinal cord, on the side opposite to that of the lesion, through the entire length of the lateral fasciculus down to the lumbar enlargement.

III. I think some explanations concerning the anatomy and pathological physiology of *secondary degenerative* or *descending scleroses*, as they still may be called, will not here

---

[1] Experiences of Ferrier, Carville and Duret.

be amiss. They are incontestably one of the principal causes of the persistence of motor impotency in the cases under consideration. In my opinion, we must also join to them the major part of *permanent contractions*, called *late contractions* (*tardive*)[1] which in these cases sooner or later take possession of the paralyzed limbs, and in a general way play a predominant rôle in the prognosis of cerebral hemorrhage.

1st. Let us first pause in face of a fact which really rules the question : cerebral lesions (*en foyer*), considered as respects their location, are not all equally able to produce consecutive sclerosis.

Thus, among these lesions, some are never followed by descending sclerosis, while others almost surely are. To this last kind belong destructive lesions, however slight, which, according to the important observation of L. Türck, involve the fasciculi of the internal capsule in their course between the lenticular and caudated ganglia, that is, along the anterior two-thirds of the capsule. On the contrary, those lesions confined to the substance of the gray cerebral masses, namely, the lenticulated and caudated ganglia and the thalami optici, produce no consecutive sclerosis.

That remarkable fact was thoroughly brought to light by L. Türck [2] in 1851. Vulpian and I have both recognized its entire exactitude in the researches which we have made together at Salpêtrière from 1861 to 1866.[3] The important works of Bouchard have equally confirmed it.[4] There are also a certain number of other facts, furnished by L. Türck, not less interesting, and of which the following is the gist :

[1] We are indebted, as is known, to Dr. Todd for having established a distinction between early and late (*précoce et tardive*) contraction in the limbs of an apoplectic. The first appears at the commencement and is nearly always transitory ; the other does not appear before the fourteenth to the thirtieth day after the attack, is situated always in the limbs of the side opposite to the lesion, and in the majority of cases is permanent.

[2] L. Türck.—Ueber secundäre Erkrankung einzelner Rückenmarksstränge und ihrer Forsetzungen zum Gehirne. Sitzungsber. der mathnatur. Classe d. K. Ak., 1851. Idem., XI. Bd., 1853.

[3] A. Vulpian.—Physiologie du système nerveux, Paris, 1866.

[4] Ch. Bouchard.— Des dégénérations secondaires de la molle épinière. In Arch. gén. de médecine, 1866.

2d. Lesions situated outside of the central masses, in the centrum ovale of Vieussens, produce descending sclerosis, provided they are not too far removed from the foot of the radiating fibres (*couronne rayonnante*).

3d. Lesions of the gray cortical substance of the hemispheres, when they are very superficial, such, for example, as those which habitually accompany meningitis, do not produce descending sclerosis.

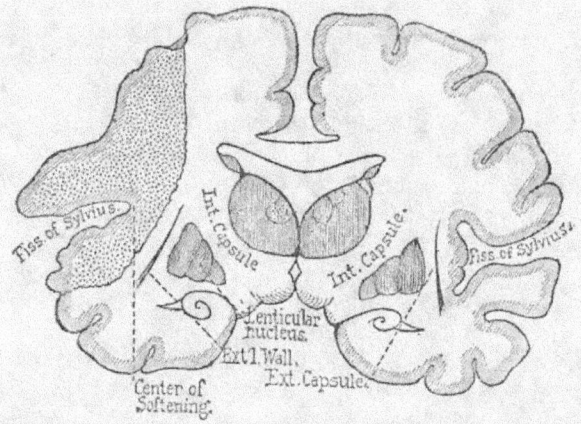

FIG. 37.—Cortical ischæmic softening without involving the central masses.

4th. On the contrary, cortical lesions which are both extended and profound, that is, involving both the gray substance and the subjacent medullary substance, as seen in cases of ischæmic softening resulting, for example, from the obliteration of a voluminous branch of the Sylvian artery (see Fig. 37)—these lesions, I say, even *when there is no participation of the central masses*, produce *in certain cases* consecutive sclerosis as marked as that which depends upon a lesion of the anterior region of the internal capsule.

Among these conditions there is one especially relating to the location of cortical lesions, which should be made particularly clear. We have observed that superficial softenings (yellow patches) occupying either the occipital lobe, the posterior parts of the temporal or sphenoidal lobe, or the anterior regions of the frontal lobe, are not succeeded by consecutive fascicular sclerosis, while on the other hand these scleroses, as a rule, follow lesions of the two ascending convolutions (ascending parietal and ascending frontal), and the contiguous parts of the parietal and frontal lobes (Fig. 38). Further on I will return more especially to this point, which I now merely mention.

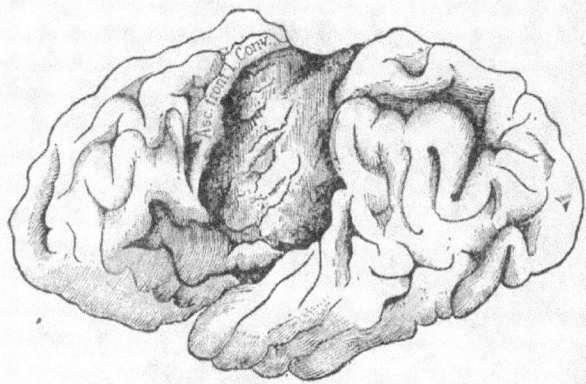

FIG. 38.—Human brain, left side ; destruction of the ascending parietal convolution and a great part of the ascending frontal convolution.

5th. In brief, the locality and extent of the lesion seem here to be the two fundamental conditions ; the nature of the lesion seems to have no marked influence. The required locality and extent being given, descending sclerosis should follow, provided the lesion is a destructive one, that is, one capable of interrupting the course of the medullary fibres. Centres of hemorrhage or softening, and simple or syphilitic encephalitis, have in this respect much the same rank. It is not the same with certain tumors which, through a long period of evolution, only crowd back or to one side the medullary elements without interrupting their continuity. This is the reason why they may exist, even in the regions above specified, unaccompanied by consecutive fascicular sclerosis.

IV. As for the anatomy of fascicular sclerosis, I refer for details to the important *mémoire* published by Bouchard. I will only remind you of some facts to which our present studies give a particular interest.

1st. I will commence by recalling that sclerosis following a lesion *(en foyer)* in the cerebral hemispheres always occupies one-half of the lateral fasciculi. It is more or less marked and more or less extensive according to the size of the fasciculus; but always extends down to the inferior end of the lumbar enlargement, never stops by the way. They are always *descending*, in the sense that, taking origin on a level with the point of lesion, they never extend except below that point; they are never found above it, towards the gray cortex. The atrophy of one or several of the convolutions, or even of the entire hemisphere, such as is seen when a central lesion *(en foyer)* is developed in very young subjects, is not necessarily the result of a sclerosis. That arises from an arrest of development which may be compared to atrophy, which, under like circumstances, is to be seen in the limbs upon the side of the body affected by hemiplegia (infantile spasmodic hemiplegia).

2d. Microscopic examination alone, in cases which have existed for some time and are rather marked, can recognize some of the most prominent characters of the alteration. Let us suppose a yellow patch, interrupting in the left hemisphere the course of the fibres of the internal capsule in its middle third. In such a case the foot of the crus cerebri of the left side will appear flatter and narrower than that of the opposite side. There will also be seen a grayish band situated upon the middle part of the peduncle,[1] which upon an antero-posterior section does not extend beyond the gray layer of Soemmering. The gray color disappears at the level of the protuberance; it is found again below, in the bulb, where it occupies the entire extent of the anterior pyramid on the side corresponding to the cerebral lesion; the affected pyramid is

---

[1] The situation occupied by that band varies according to the location of the central lesion; it is nearer the internal border of the foot of the peduncle in proportion as the lesion of the capsule is situated anteriorly.

narrowed and flattened; lower down, the teeth of the bulbular decussation show more distinctly than in the normal condition by reason of the contrast which exists between the sound and diseased sides. Below the decussation it is in the opposite side of the spinal cord (opposite to the affected hemisphere), in the lateral fasciculus, that the sclerosis should be sought for; the alteration is in the form of a triangular space, of gray color, situated immediately external and anterior to the corresponding posterior gray cornu, the area of which lessens in proportion as the sections are made lower down on the cord.

3d. Microscopic studies, made upon sections properly hardened and prepared, greatly contribute to our knowledge. In the first place, they furnish the means for locating more exactly the topography of the lesion, and to make known, in the spinal cord, for example, the precise limitation of the area in the lateral fasciculus. The other white fasciculi and the gray cornua remain entirely unchanged. It is to be noticed, at the same time, that the roots of the nerves, anterior and posterior, as well as the meninges, exhibit no trace of alteration.

Lastly, the microscope makes known also the nature of the morbid process, and furnishes proof of a gray induration—a sclerosis which differs in no essential particular from that observed in cases of primitive fascicular sclerosis.[1]

4th. Here is the place to call attention to the analogies which exist in an anatomico-pathological point of view between consecutive fascicular sclerosis, of cerebral origin, and those primitive and symmetrical fascicular scleroses of the lateral fasciculi which I last year described in connection with spinal muscular atrophy (*amyotrophics spinales*).

These analogies are considerable, since the same alteration (gray induration) is in both cases located in the same tissue. But there are also variations worthy of notice; thus, in primitive sclerosis the fascicular lesions are necessarily double, that

---

[1] Those cases where the extension of the lesion exceeds its habitual limits, the invasion, for example, of the anterior gray cornua, which will be considered farther on, are certainly among the most decisive arguments which can be employed to establish the irritative nature of the morbid process.

is, they occupy the lateral fasciculi of both sides simultaneously, instead of one side only, as is always the case in consecutive sclerosis, when the lesion from which it arises is unilateral. I will also add that it is very much less extended
transversely, and there is reason to believe, therefore, that
beyond the cerebro-spinal or pyramidal fibres, which are the
only ones affected in consecutive sclerosis, primitive sclero-

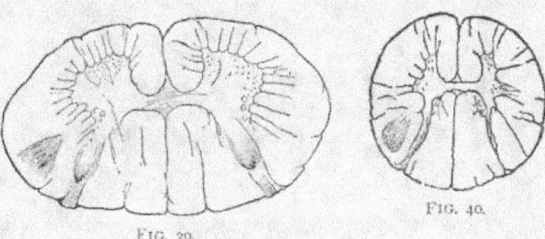

FIG. 39.

FIG. 40.

FIG. 39.—Transverse section of the spinal cord in a case of consecutive lateral fascicular sclerosis ; from softening of the optico-striated bodies and the internal capsule.
(Cervical region.)
FIG. 40.—Transverse section of the spinal cord in a case of consecutive lateral
fascicular sclerosis. (Dorsal region.)

sis invades also the spinal fibres of the lateral fasciculus (compare Figs. 39, 40, and 41, and Figs. 42, 43, and 44).

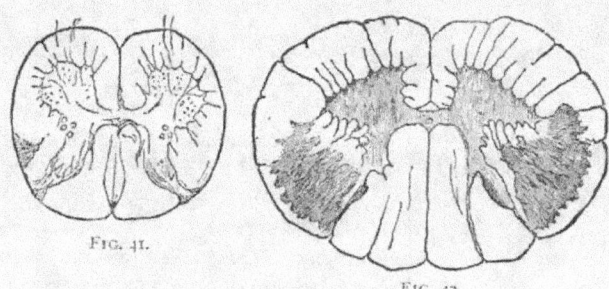

FIG. 41.

FIG. 42.

FIG. 41.—Transverse section of the spinal cord in a case of consecutive lateral
fascicular sclerosis. (Lumbar region.)
FIG. 42.—Transverse section of the spinal cord in a case of primitive lateral
fascicular sclerosis. (Middle portion of cervical enlargement.)

Finally, primitive sclerosis has a great tendency to extend
to the neighboring spinal regions, to the white fasciculi, and

especially the anterior cornua of the gray substance, which is not the rule in the consecutive form.[1]

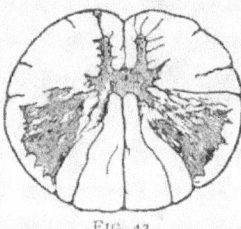 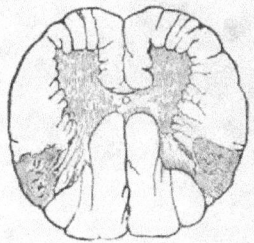

FIG. 43.

FIG. 44.

FIG. 43.—Transverse section of the spinal cord in a case of primitive lateral fascicular sclerosis.   (Middle of dorsal region.)

FIG. 44.—Transverse section of the spinal cord in a case of primitive lateral fascicular sclerosis.   (Middle of lumbar enlargement.)

---

[1] Here are some more precise details relative to the anatomical differences existing between consecutive lateral sclerosis and primitive lateral sclerosis, amyotrophic.   They are examinations made upon hardened transverse sections, where, even in the bulb, secondary sclerosis has involved nearly all the fibres of the anterior pyramid, and in the spinal cord the lesion occupies only a comparatively narrow space in the lateral fasciculus.   Upon a transverse section made at the cervical enlargement, the lesion is seen as a triangle with very clearly defined borders, the apex of which is directed inward toward the angle which separates the anterior from the posterior gray cornua, the base a little rounded, does not extend to the circumference of the cord, neither does it involve the antero-external border of the posterior cornu (Fig. 39).   In the dorsal region the sclerotic portion progressively diminishes in diameter and tends to resume an oval form (Fig. 40). Finally, in the lumbar enlargement (Fig. 41), it resumes as in the cervical region, a sort of triangle, but in this locality the base of the triangle is quite superficial, next to the pia mater.

In primitive lateral sclerosis, the sclerotic zone occupies in a general way the same region as does consecutive sclerosis, but its area is much greater.   Thus, anteriorly, the lesion tends to invade the anterior radiating zones, and internally it extends so as to come in contact with the nerve-fibres (perhaps sensitive) which constitute the profound part of the lateral fasciculi (see Figs. 42, 43, 44).   It must be added that here the borders of the lesions become ill-defined.   In some cases they seem to be confounded with the gray substance.   It is known that the gray substance is regularly invaded by sclerotic alterations in cases of lateral amyotrophic sclerosis, whereas it is very exceptional in consecutive sclerosis from cerebral cause.

From the preceding considerations there is reason to think that consecutive sclerosis affects only one part of the nerve-fibres which compose the lateral fasciculi, namely, the cerebro-spinal fibres; whereas, in primitive sclerosis, it invades

There is, however, a chapter of exceptions which in this connection is particularly interesting.

IV. The facts gathered in the course of the preceding *exposé* enable us to justify the proposition with which this chapter commenced. We have established in an anatomical point of view that there exists a very considerable analogy between primitive and consecutive forms of lateral fascicular sclerosis. That assimilation can be followed upon the clinical field. It is known, indeed, that motor loss, contraction of the limbs, at first transient, then permanent, with spontaneous or provoked trepidation, etc., provide a symptomatic group which reveals during life the existence of primitive fascicular spinal sclerosis, that is, independent of any cerebral lesion. Now all the essential characters of these symptoms are reproduced in sclerosis arising from a lesion in the brain, the clinical picture, in fact, of common permanent hemiplegia. It may be said, then, that there exists a relation between the phenomenon of " permanent contraction " and " lateral sclerosis," the physiological reason of which at present completely eludes us, but the reality of which is nevertheless established by a great number of observations.[1]

In my opinion, it is not the retraction of the cerebral cicatrix, as Todd would hold, nor yet encephalitis supervening from proximity to the lesion, as very many authors at present maintain, which can explain the apparition of those contractions in hemiplegias called tardy (*tardive*) ; on the contrary, it is more reasonable to attribute it to a chronic myelitis in the lateral fasciculus resulting from the cerebral lesion. I will avoid discussion, and once more refer you to the work already cited of Bouchard, in which will be found all the proofs that can be adduced in favor of my opinion.

Consecutive sclerosis resulting from cerebral lesion ac-

the entire lateral system, including not only the cerebro-spinal and pyramidal fibres, but also those fibres which both commence and terminate in the spinal cord—those *fibres properly called spinal fibres.*

[1] Permanent contraction of the limbs, as is seen in other complaints, such as hysteria, may exist without lateral spinal sclerosis ; but when that lesion exists, permanent contraction is an habitual symptom.

9

quires, after a given time, a kind of independent existence, automatic; this is evinced by special symptoms. By reason of this autonomy the lesion may happen to extend beyond the limits habitually assigned to it in the lateral fasciculus, and invade the adjacent parts of the spinal cord, the substance of the gray cornua, for example; in such cases it is comprehensible that important modifications may occur in the symptomatic tableau; thus, the muscles of the paralyzed limbs, which in permanent hemiplegia ordinarily preserve their normal texture for a long time, and but slowly emaciate, are subject, in certain cases, to a degenerative atrophy, more or less rapid, at the same time that the rigidity of the contraction gives way to renewed flaccidity. In several examples of this kind, Pierret and I have demonstrated, in addition to the classic lateral sclerosis, a lesion of the anterior gray cornu of the same side, including the destruction of the large nerve-cells of that region. The invasion of the posterior gray cornu might in like manner explain the appearance of certain partial anæsthesia in common hemiplegia. Lastly, the extension of the initiative process, whether along the whole course of the lateral fasciculus of the corresponding side, or be it of the lateral fasciculus of the opposite side, would doubtless explain the fact that, contrary to common observation, the contraction of the lower limb is at some one period considerably greater, or sometimes extends to the opposite limb.[1]

V. To the present I have only occupied myself with fascicular sclerosis arising from lesion of the central cerebral masses. I now wish to give a moment to those produced by lesions of the cortex. So far as concerns the affection of the spine or the bulb, lateral sclerosis, from lesions of the central masses, in no way differs from that following lesions of the cortex. The special conditions of development constitute all the difference, and this calls for new details.

You remember how you have been led to admit, on the grounds of a very probable hypothesis, the existence of *di-*

[1] In this connection see Bastian—Paralysis from Brain Diseases, etc., p. 141. London, 1875.

rect peduncular fibres—that is, those which, after leaving the
foot of the peduncle, traverse the internal capsule without
entering the gray ganglia of the central masses, and consequently do not stop until they reach the gray cortical substance; besides the arguments already employed, some facts
of experimentation can be cited in favor of the existence of
such fibres, even with animals of low scale, the rabbit for example. Thus in the experiments already noticed of Gudden,[1]
made upon very young animals, it is seen that eight months
after the removal of the anterior part of a hemisphere, the
central masses, thalami optici, and corpora striata being untouched, the internal capsule of the corresponding side atro-
phies in a remarkable manner. It is clear that such atrophy
would not occur if the internal capsule, as some anatomists
hold, were exclusively composed of *indirect peduncular fibres*,
—that is, of fibres terminating in the substance of the central
gray ganglia.

Chance brought to the notice of Carville and Duret[2] a
lesion in a dog which had destroyed all the white substance
of the frontal portion of a lobe without directly affecting the
central gray ganglia or the internal capsule. In this case
there was a very marked atrophy of the foot of the peduncle,
the protuberance, and of the pyramidal bulb of the side corresponding to the cerebral lesion.

The reality of these direct peduncular fibres in man seems
in its turn to be proven by the production of the secondary
degenerations which, as we have said, are a result of extensive and deep lesions of the gray cortical substance.

Do these direct peduncular fibres, after their disappearance
in the diverging fibres, spread indifferently to all parts of the
hemisphere, or are they assigned to special departments of
the gray cortex? The facts which I have collected towards
the study of that question plead in favor of the last hypothesis. These observations, collected for me at the Hospital of
Saltpêtrière during the last fifteen years, relate to cases of

---

[1] Archiv für Psychiatrie, Bd. II., 1870, pl. VIII.
[2] Archives de physiologie, 1875.

long-standing ischæmic softening.[1]   The lesions in these cases
appeared as *yellow patches* of variable size, extending more
or less deeply into the subjacent white substance and occupying the most diverse regions of the surface of the hemispheres.   In all the cases it is expressly mentioned that the
softenings had left the central masses, thalami optici, caudated and lenticular ganglia, and internal capsule, entirely
untouched.   My observations may be divided into two
groups.

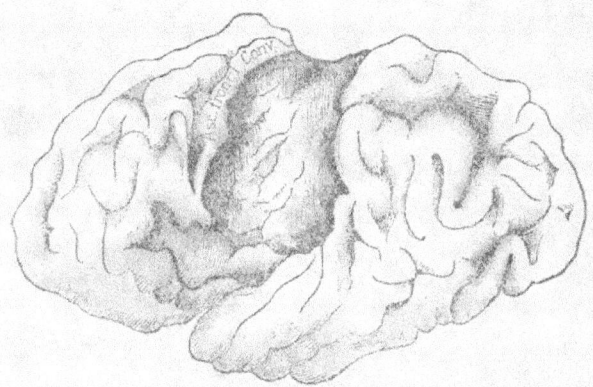

Fig. 45.—Human brain, left side ; destruction of the ascending parietal convolution and a great part of the ascending frontal convolution.

The first includes those cases where no permanent hemiplegia existed during life, and where autopsy discovered no
consecutive degeneration.   In all these cases the convolutions fed by the Sylvian artery, and especially the ascending
frontal and parietal convolutions, had remained unharmed.
The yellow patch occupied one of the following regions,
namely, some part of the sphenoidal lobes, the quadrilateral
lobule, the cuneus, one or both of the occipital lobes, and a
region ranging over the anterior two-thirds of the frontal
lobes.

[1] The most of these observations are accompanied by designs made from nature ;
it can be understood that the place and extent of the lesion are thus more exactly
located, and consequently the ordinary insufficiency of description is avoided.

In all cases of the second group, there had been, on the contrary, a permanent hemiplegia, and the consecutive sclerosis was perfectly marked. The distinguishing feature of these cases was, that the lesion always involved more or less one or the other of the ascending frontal or parietal convolutions, chiefly in their superior half, and often both of the convolutions were at the same time affected ; besides, the regions nearest to the frontal and parietal convolutions generally participated. The design which I place before you is a very marked example (Fig. 45).

From the preceding, as I before said, it would seem that secondary sclerosis, resulting from destructive lesions of the cerebral cortex, are subordinate to location. I will add, in conclusion, that those portions of the cortex a lesion of which determines secondary degenerations exclusively, correspond to those parts which experimentation with the monkey has designated as the psycho-motor centres. They are the same also where the gray cortical substance contains the largest pyramidal cells.

I have brought into relief an important fact, which should be utilized in the study of localization in the cerebral cortex ; a difficult study which we will attempt in our next lectures.

www.ingramcontent.com/pod-product-compliance
Lightning Source LLC
Chambersburg PA
CBHW081259170526
45165CB00011B/3354